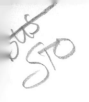
The
Sports Medicine Guide For
# The Everyday Athlete

By
# Thomas W. Harris, M.D.

Tomlin International
La Jolla

*This book is dedicated to*
the Everyday Athlete

# Acknowledgements

In keeping with the Sports Medicine team approach, I could not have completed this book without the efforts of the other contributors. Sections of this book deserve special acknowledgements.

Chapters three and four, *Training and Conditioning* and *Individual Training Program* include the input of Russ Sinclair. Russ is an exercise physiologist who specializes in exercise therapy. Chapter four includes exercises demonstrated by Russ and Mary Faith. I had the privilege of sitting in the director's chair and made director's comments during the photo sessions. Thanks to the patience and professionalism of the photographer, Roger Andrews, the results are excellent.

Chapter eight, *Focus on the Foot*, was a combined effort of Joe Ellis, D.P.M. and myself. Dr. Ellis, a marathon runner and triathlete, is well known for his expertise in sports-related foot problems.

Chapter sixteen, *Nutrition—Food, Fuel and Fluids*, includes the input of Francis Nettl, M.D., M.P.H., a world class athlete himself (plus being a world class person and physician.) Dr. Nettl had great input in the area of anabolic steroids.

Nobody deserves more recognition than my wife, Linda, who spent untold hours toiling over this manuscript in an editing capacity.

Thanks also to:

Steve Cook for his exceptional artwork.

Catherine Hansson for her patience and talent in making my vision for the cover a reality.

The Athletic Orthopedic Institute—especially the administrator Lenny Kurtz, M.S., A.T.C. Their hard work, loyalty and compassion are commendable and I'm proud to have them on my team.

My friend, Tom House, Ph.D., pitching coach for the Texas Rangers—shown in action later in this book.

Athletic Trainers such as Jim Hammond, A.T.C., Al Esquivel, A.T.C., and Linda Greer, A.T.C., are there, on the field and behind the scenes working hard to make it all work. Also Ed Ayub, M.S.P.T., therapist and Head Trainer for the U.S. Rugby Team.

Physical therapists such as Pat Yavorsky, R.P.T., Kathy Grace, R.P.T., and Virginia Greg, R.P.T., A.T.C. Also the staffs of the Harbor View Medical Center's Physical Therapy Department, Orthopedic and Sport Physical Therapy, La Jolla Sports Therapy and Sports and Orthopedic Physical Therapy Specialists.

The U.S. Ski Team's coaches, trainers and staff—especially Topper Hagerman, Ph.D., and John Atkins, A.T.C.

Bob Babbitt—editor of Competitor Magazine and first class athlete.

The staff of Harbor View Medical Center.

The Chart House Running Team and the San Diego Track Club—devoted athletes who have made fitness part of their everyday lives.

# CONTENTS

# INTRODUCTION

## WHO IS THE EVERYDAY ATHLETE?

Every person is a potential Everyday Athlete. People just like you and me, people from two to 92, from nine months to 90 years. The Everyday Athlete is a person who cares about his or her health and who wants to feel better, look better, live longer, be more mentally alert—in other words, have a longer, better, more satisfying life.

In this book I present guidelines for you to achieve just that. Understand your body. Understand how it gets injured and understand how to get it in shape from scratch. Use the guidelines in this book; practice the principles and make it an enjoyable part of your everyday life and you will become an Everyday Athlete.

The fitness boom has almost been a fitness bust, because of the high injury rate associated with exercise. Over the last twenty years, we have become aware of a need for fitness in order to improve the quality of life and decrease heart disease, but we did not know how to get there. With injury rates up to 70 percent in people doing exercise programs, you can see that the fitness boom has not entirely succeeded.

How did we get where we are? Around the turn of the century, people in our society did not concern themselves with fitness because just about everybody was fit. Eighty percent of the population walked four to five hours a day. Back then, fitness was a part of the everyday lifestyle. Most people were Everyday Athletes—they just didn't know it. Then over the next twenty years, we changed from a walking society to a sitting society. At the same time, the quality of nutrition deteriorated as well. If you combine poor nutrition with lack of exercise and poor posture, you're destined to end up with a generation of people with poor health conditions.

Around 1965, 80% of the population walked for only five minutes a day. Over 80% of the population spent their working hours sitting down. Over the years, cardiovascular disease had increased from nine to 53%!

The need to emphasize the study of Sports Medicine soon became apparent. And, through this interest, we discovered how to actually improve health and well-being through exercise—and do it injury-free, to boot. Since then, we have found that exercise and an improvement in nutrition can significantly decrease the incidence of heart disease.

Being an Everyday Athlete does not mean that you have to work out every day. You make the principles a part of your everyday life. And just because you were once injured in exercise does not mean you are out of the fitness game. Make a comeback. But do it right this time. Be a winning player in the fitness game.

First, understand the basics of how the body works. Understand what makes a safe training and conditioning program—ways that we can achieve the goals of the Everyday Athlete with our urban lifestyle and busy schedules.

Gone are the days when people who exercised were called "exercise freaks," or people who cared about what they ate were called "health food fanatics." In today's society, with mass communication, education and new research available, most people are interested in improving their health and maintaining it as well.

This book is designed to help you better understand your body, how it works, how and why to exercise it, how it is injured and how to prevent those injuries.

The athlete of today is much more sophisticated than ever before about such things as fitness, nutrition and the availability of professional help. This highly-informed individual expects that the professional Sports Medicine team will offer the finest, most advanced medical program available today. The more sophisticated Sports Medicine teams are important players in the recreational athlete's total athletic program. They are keenly aware that the injured athlete has to get back into action as quickly as possible. The Everyday Athlete wants the same kind of high tech, professional help that the pros receive. A host of these very aware athletes find their way to our centers. They come prepared to learn about their injuries and apply the latest methods of Sports Medicine, taking advantage of the finest, most comprehensive care and education available in the world. They already have a basic understanding of the Sports Medicine team and expect the most sophisticated help. The orthopedic surgeon, the trainer and the coach, the physical therapist, the family doctor and the exercise physiologist are some of the highly-trained specialists who make certain the recreational athlete gets the very best care.

Having worked with thousands of athletes through the years, I have found that the single most important thing is to educate people about injury. If the patient is well informed and knowledgeable, then the treatment, rehabilitation and prevention battles are half won. It is also beneficial for an athlete to have an understanding of the vital roles of those working with him or her. A well-informed athlete sustained by a professional, well-informed support team ensures the best treatment.

"What caused the injury?"
"What is the actual injury?"
"How can it be treated?"
"When can I safely go back to sports?"
"What are the long-term effects of this injury?"
"What can I do to prevent this from happening again?"
"What kind of exercise program should I use in my fitness and prevention program?"

These are logical questions that any athlete deserves to ask about his or her own medical problem, and these are some of the questions which will be addressed in this book. There are a number of excellent textbooks about Sports Medicine, but most are written to educate the professionals: doctors, trainers, therapists, etc. This book is not meant to be a medical text; it was written to educate the everyday or potential Everyday Athlete about his or her body as it relates to sports readiness and to offer a view of state-of-the-art medical and therapeutic care in Sports Medicine.

There are methods employed by the medical team that support the world class athlete. These same methods are readily available to the non-professional as well. It is a matter of knowing what to do and where to go. Some aspects of the scope of sports readiness and rehabilitation can be self-taught or at least understood well enough so that when the athlete does seek professional help, the groundwork is already in place.

The study of Sports Medicine has certainly come of age. There is an incredible increase in participation and interest in the subject by athletes and physicians alike. Almost daily, 50 percent of the population in America participates in some form of athletic activity. Roughly 70 percent of the population is either a spectator or a participant in sports.

This has brought about an increased interest in preventive treatment and rehabilitation, and the field of Sports Medicine is exploding. One of the main reasons for the great success in this area of medicine is the enthusiastic participation of the injured athlete and the healthy athlete as well. And it goes without saying that the more these athletes know and understand, the better patients they become. In reality, the athlete wants to be healthy, and that is why he or she takes a keen interest in the prevention and treatment phase of their programs.

Regular athletic activity in itself can be preventive medicine by relieving stress and fighting depression, heart disease and obesity, but only if injury is avoided or properly treated. Many enthusiastic fitness programs have fallen into disfavor because of the high injury rates. This is especially so among the beginning or starting-over athletes, over thirty, who simply were not properly introduced to the correct manner of starting a fitness program.

Focusing on individual goals like decreasing stress, weight loss or decreasing heart disease, while neglecting any attention to the body's structure, is a major weakness in many fitness and sports programs. It does no good to rush into a weight loss program that ignores proper fitness and training. When attention is paid to all aspects of fitness, training and conditioning, it makes for a successful Sports Medicine program.

It is the health professionals who must properly instruct this rising number of over-thirty athletes. A revolution in sports has taken place in that the schools are no longer the centers for athletics; the center has shifted to the ski slopes, jogging trails, health clubs, etc., including a vast segment of middle-aged men and women. Injury prevention is no longer only the concern of the coach or the orthopedist, now the family doctor and the heart specialist must be just as concerned with preventing injuries as the fitness instructor. No longer is the player only the young and vigorous, in the very prime of physical strength and endurance. Millions of over-thirty athletes have a driving desire to maintain or regain the fitness and endurance they once had in school.

Some school programs require pre-participation examinations by physicians and other professionals for an age group with much lower risk of injury, while the older participant, who lacks good coordination and flexibility, rushes into a sport with little thought to his or her physical ability to withstand the perils of the potential danger to the body. A good example of this is the middle-aged executive who, having done little, if any, exercise for the past 15 years, decides to take up a sport. With no professional guidance or evaluation, these athletes usually end up with as much as a 70 percent injury rate...and of course, quit exercising. This type of person, who can best afford a professional program of instruction and least afford the time off work, does not realize how important preparation and professional help can be.

Another revolution in sports has been the increasing participation of women. For instance, women's participation in intercollegiate sports has increased fivefold in the last decade. There are certain unique characteristics of the female which should be considered by the Sports Medicine specialist. There are, for example, strength differences between her and her counterpart which take place after puberty. Other unique factors of the female athlete that should be considered are pelvic size, gait differences, possible pregnancy, as well as varied hormonal differences. Unless otherwise stated, the principles of the book are meant to apply to the male and female. Properly conditioned female athletes have injury rates equal to males under similar sports conditions. Training studies have shown that women exhibit equal percentages of improvement in areas such as coordination, strength and endurance if exposed to similar exercise of equal frequency, intensity and duration. Particular conditions which apply specifically to the male or female will be addressed appropriately throughout the book.

I hope you enjoy reading the material as much as I have enjoyed writing it. Remember, It's **fun to be fit**. Whenever you're fit, you are bound to **have a good day**.

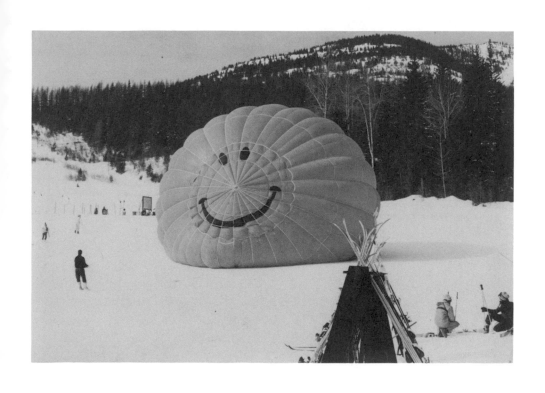

# Framework for Motion

# Framework for Motion

"The head bone's connected to the—neck bone, the neck bone's connected to the—shoulder bone..." Remember that oldy?

If you heard me sing this you would really understand one meaning of out of tune and would quickly tune me out. But fortunately you don't have to listen to me sing in order to understand more of what makes our amazing bodies work so that we can tune in to them, tone them up and have them work harmoniously. Just read along and follow the bouncing ball.

## YOUR AMAZING BODY

The human body is truly amazing. Under normal conditions, the body is able to heal itself, combat infection and adapt to unusual environments and trauma. The body has a built-in alarm system which is triggered when something goes wrong. Some of the warning signals are aches, pains, headaches, dizziness, and nausea. When an athlete experiences a new or consistent pain, it's a warning. He or she should listen to their body and seek assistance from their medical team. Caught early, treatment may consist of simply taping by the trainer, a flexibility and strengthening program with the physical therapist, or perhaps just a new pair of not-so-broken-down running shoes. If, however, the warning signals are ignored and the athlete "works through the pain," he or she could end up "on the bench" for weeks or months at a time, and might even need surgery.

## THE SKELETAL SYSTEM

The skeletal system is a framework held up by the muscle system. Together, they are called the *musculoskeletal system*, which is responsible for body movement. The skeleton serves three functions: it provides a rigid framework for the muscles to attach to, it helps protect the internal organs and it produces red and white blood cells in the bone marrow.

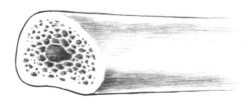

*Cross section of bone showing cortex and marrow*

## JOINTS OF THE BODY

A *joint* is the site where two or more bones join together, whether or not there is movement between them. There are joints which don't move—for example, the growth plates in children. However, we will discuss only two types of joints. The first type has little movement and is joined by a thick, fibrous tissue (or *fibrocartilage*). Examples are the discs between the bodies of the vertebra. The other type of joints, the *synovial joints*, has the maximal amount of movement. Examples of these are the knee joints, finger joints, the elbow, the shoulder and the ankle joints. Most of our focus will be on the anatomy and function of synovial joints.

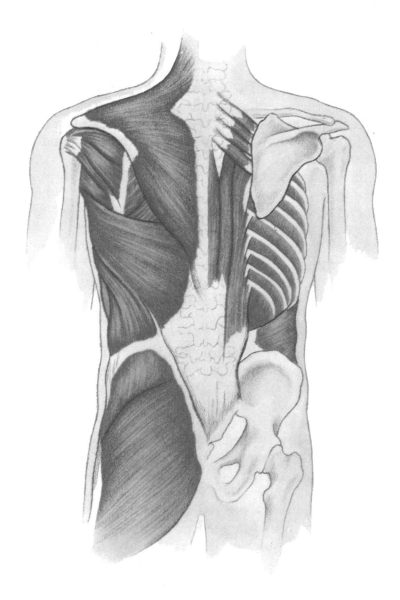

*Diagram of the back showing the muscle attachments and the anatomical relationships.*

In the synovial joint, the bony surfaces are covered with a tough padding called *cartilage*. There is a sac surrounding each synovial joint called the *capsule*. A thin inner lining of the capsule, the *synovium*, secretes the lubricating fluid called *synovial fluid*.

## LIGAMENTS

Joints are held in place by *ligaments*. Ligaments are strong, fibrous bands of collagen which have very little elasticity but are pliable. They reinforce the capsule and give stability to the joint. Ligaments attach from bone to bone between the two bone ends, giving static strength to the joint. In other words, the ligaments hold the joint together. If ligaments are torn or stretched, an unstable joint can result.

The thicker the ligaments are, the stronger they are and the better they support the joint from coming apart. A sprain happens when the joint is forced to move in an abnormal direction and the force exceeds the strength of the ligament. A *sprain* is a tear in the ligament, either a minor or a complete tear.

Most joints function much like a hinge to allow movement in the bony framework and, like a hinge, restrict movement to a given distance, or *range of motion* (ROM). Some joints function like a "ball-in-socket," and allow a greater ROM (shoulder, hip). The ROM of all joints is restricted by the capsule and ligaments. When a joint bends beyond its capacity (ROM), immediate damage results. For example, a strain/sprain injury can result in torn ligaments and muscle attachments, and/or ruptured synovial sacs.

Once a joint is damaged, it can become unstable and unable to remain in its intended position. It can become loose, weak and difficult to control, unable to support its ordinary weight-load.

A damaged joint often becomes the site of traumatic arthritis, recognizable by swelling and by chronically painful movement.

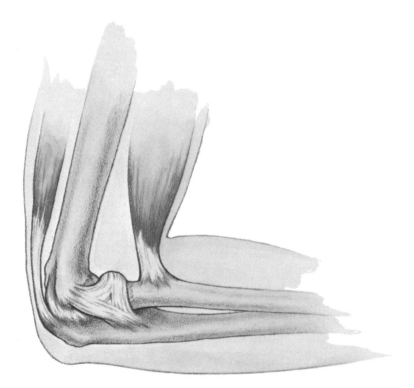

*This illustration of the elbow joint shows the ligamentous structures laterally. The biceps muscle with its tendon attachment to the radius contracts, flexing the elbow. The triceps and triceps tendon attachment posterially contracts, extending the elbow.*

## THE MUSCLES

There are three types of muscle tissue in your body: voluntary muscles, involuntary muscles and the heart muscle.

*Voluntary muscles* are the muscles we can move at will. They are the muscles that move the joints. *Involuntary muscles* are the smooth muscles that cause movement in the glands, skin and organs—especially the stomach and intestines. The *heart muscle*, a special blend of muscle fibers that pumps the blood throughout our bodies, is an involuntary muscle.

Voluntary muscles act like the strings of the puppeteer, pulleys which move our limbs and spine in various directions. They have a broad attachment into the shaft or end of the bone they serve and, on the opposite end, insert into another bone which may be more fixed.

Contracting muscle fibers pull the bone in a given direction. While this appears as a single movement, for every muscle contraction there must be a simultaneous relaxation of the muscle with which it works—synergistically—in a rhythmic harmony of contraction/relaxation.

It's important that your muscles work together and that their timing is correct. This interaction between the nervous system and the muscles is called *coordination*. For example, several muscle groups cooperate to permit you to raise your arm above your head. One group takes the arm to a certain height and releases it, when another group takes over. This process is repeated until your arm is over your head. This relay effort—a series of simultaneous contractions and relaxations—is a classic example of *synergistic action*. Plainly, the inability to move a part to its fullest limit may be caused by the failure of one or more muscle groups to contract or relax in harmony.

Just as strength, endurance and flexibility can be improved with training, coordination can also be improved. With proper, specific training, the efficiency of the nerve pathway can be improved.

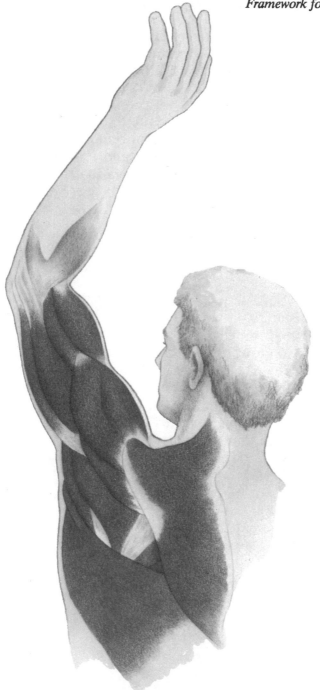

*Complex integration of muscle and nerve activity is needed to raise the arm over the head.*

We have all heard the saying, "You've got to tone up those muscles." But do we actually know what that means? Healthful muscle firmness is called "tone." A body out of shape, weak and unwilling to work, lacks the "tone" necessary to provide erectness of posture and the energy to accomplish the ordinary work requirements of daily life.

So you see, it is all interrelated. The skeletal system is supported by the muscle system and joints are held in place by ligaments that need to be strong. Muscles need to have strength, tone, endurance and flexibility and the nerve pathways need to function unimpaired so that they all work in harmony.

There is little doubt that everyone listens to the radio on occasion. Have you ever been kicking-back on the beach and bumped the radio by accident only to have the station you were listening to replaced by massive static and what sounds like four high-pitched mariachis all singing and laughing at the same time? Or have you ever played an old piano only to find that C sounds like D and B sounds like something you'd use to call your dog? Well, it appears that both your radio and your piano are out of tune. The radio needs to be tuned in and the piano needs to be tuned up. And your body? As you might have guessed, **STAYING TUNED AND TONED IS THE NAME OF THE GAME.**

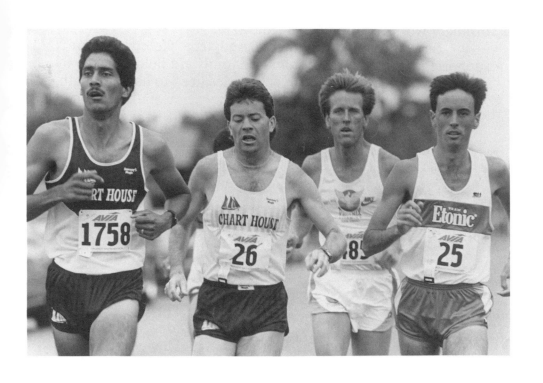

**Chapter Two**
# Preparing Your Body

# Preparing Your Body

When someone tells you that they are fit, what exactly does that mean? That they're "buffed out to the max" and have such large biceps that they make Sylvester Stallone look like Pee Wee Herman? That they can easily run 10 miles without even breathing hard or breaking a sweat? Or that they are so limber and flexible that even Gumby looks stiff by comparison? No. Fitness is much more, something that's not quite that easy to put a finger on.

## FITNESS

Fitness can be defined in two ways: Cardiovascular respiratory fitness and musculoskeletal fitness.

*Cardiovascular respiratory fitness* is efficient transportation and utilization of essential oxygen and nutrients to the tissues of the body. A well-conditioned cardiovascular system enables the body to deliver sufficient blood-containing oxygen and nutrients to the working muscles and, at the same time, improve the muscle capacity to use the extra oxygen. This is also called *aerobic fitness*.

*Musculoskeletal fitness* is best described as the body's ability to move at a desired level of exercise without causing injury to the muscles, tendons, ligaments, bones and joints. This involves coordination, strength, flexibility and posture.

## THE CARDIOVASCULAR RESPIRATORY SYSTEM

To understand cardiovascular respiratory fitness, you have to know how the system works. The heart muscle is constantly working, contracting and relaxing to pump blood in and out of the lungs and to the tissues of the body through the arteries, veins and capillaries. In the lungs, oxygen is absorbed into the blood and carbon dioxide is expelled.

Oxygen is carried by hemoglobin through the bloodstream and into the cells of your body. The red cells go back to the heart and are then pumped through the heart and out through the lungs, where they are reoxygenated.

During the first one or two minutes of exercise, before the heart has pumped enough oxygenated blood to the working muscles, the muscles are powered by energy produced by reactions that don't require oxygen (or *anaerobic reactions*). At this point, in order for the muscles to continue with the exercise, the body must furnish them with a continuous supply of oxygen. This is called *aerobic exercise*. The more efficiently this is done, the better the aerobic fitness (or cardiovascular respiration fitness). When the aerobic reactions cannot keep pace with the level of exercise, the body tires.

# Lungs

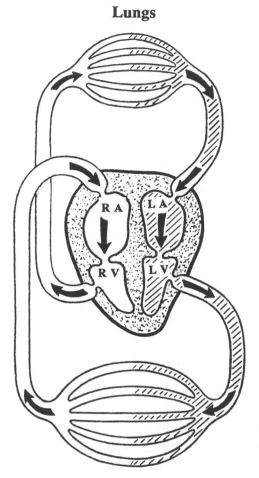

# Body Tissues

*Circulation. Blood is pumped from the heart out of the left ventricle into the aorta and from there it goes out to the tissues of the body. After the oxygen has been used, the blood then returns by the veins to the heart. It enters the heart through the right atrium, where it is then sent to the right ventricle and out into the lungs. There the blood is oxygenated and then returns from the lungs back into the left atrium to the left ventricle and back out into the body.*

How do the muscles use oxygen to produce energy? Muscles use oxygen to consume glycogen and fat to produce energy.

---

**WINNING FORMULA**
*M (Muscle) + G (Glycogen) and F (Fat) = E (Energy)*

---

When there is not enough $O_2$ present, glycogen is broken down to *lactic acid*. As lactic acid builds up in the muscles and overflows into the bloodstream, we feel fatigued. The muscle contractions slow down as the level of lactic acid builds up and eventually stop altogether. Pain and cramping may occur at this point. Anaerobic exercise can only be tolerated for a short period of time, although the well-conditioned athlete can tolerate it longer. Interval training, in the pool, on the track or on the bike is a way athletes train themselves to be able to handle the pain of going anaerobic. When triathlete Mark Allen races, he tries to go out as hard as he can as quickly as he can. The idea is to become anaerobic and to force his competitors to go anaerobic, too. Because of his exceptional training and conditioning, he feels he is able to do this longer than the other guys—and win.

In the running, triathlon and cycling world, many athletes refer to the lactic acid buildup stage as "entering the lactic acid hotel." When exercise is slowed down, the oxygen in the blood can catch up with the oxygen debt, breaking down the lactic acid to $CO_2$ and $H_2O$ to be exhaled out the lungs. When exercising aerobically, you are continuously supplying $O_2$— "Paying cash." The better your aerobic fitness, the more cash you have. On the other hand, *anaerobic exercise* is operated with an $O_2$ credit card that has a very definite limit. When you reach your credit limit, you have to pay up before you can move on. Athletes who have trained hard anaerobically have a greater credit limit—Mark Allen, for instance. The guy with the biggest credit card limit wins!

Anaerobic metabolism comes into play when energy is needed for achievements such as sprinting or lifting. Activity lasting for longer than about two minutes **must use** $O_2$ or *aerobic metabolism*.

## CHANGES THAT OCCUR WITH EXERCISE

Muscle metabolism can be significantly affected by exercise. For instance, the capacity for the muscle to utilize $O_2$ and fuel is improved by appropriate exercise. Enzyme activity is increased and the muscle can store more fuel. Less lactic acid is produced by trained muscles when undergoing moderate exercise because less glycogen is burned. With training, when less glycogen is burned with muscle contraction, less lactic acid is produced and therefore endurance improves. More fat is burned as muscle fibers hypertrophy (enlarge). Well conditioned muscles are better able to extract $O_2$ from the blood, so they require less blood supply.

It has been shown in the lab that the transmission of nerve impulses occurs more efficiently in trained versus untrained muscles, and the overall quality of nerve-muscle performance is improved.

With proper exercise, the heart becomes stronger and works more efficiently. The heart muscle uses energy more efficiently as well. At rest, the pulse is slower in trained versus untrained persons. While the heart beats fewer times per minute at rest, it delivers a greater volume of blood with each stroke (stroke volume) as a result of conditioning. During exercise the heart works more efficiently, requiring less effort to deliver greater volume. Blood pressure is lowered with conditioning, which means that the heart does not have to work as hard to pump the blood.

The level of efficiency at which your body can perform these functions measures your cardiovascular respiratory fitness. One way to measure this fitness is to monitor aerobic fitness. How much oxygen do you use per minute? The more oxygen you use per minute, the better condition you are in—from a cardiovascular respiratory standpoint. This simply means that if the heart and lungs can supply a large amount of oxygen to the tissues, you can go farther and faster before fatigue sets in.

The maximum oxygen consumption per minute is sometimes referred to as the *VO₂ Max*. This VO₂ Max is often computed by endurance athletes. The higher the number of your

$VO_2$ Max, the greater your cardiovascular respiratory fitness. $VO_2$ Max can be improved up to 25% with a proper training and conditioning program.

**In summary, the benefits of training are:**

1. **The utilization and distribution of fuel is more efficient.**
2. **Endurance is improved, with delayed fatigue.**
3. **Muscle fibers hypertrophy, giving larger muscle volume.**
4. **More fat is burned as muscle mass increases.**
5. **Nerve stimulus to muscle becomes more efficient.**

## THE EFFECT OF PROPER CONDITIONING ON HEALTH

Cardiovascular respiratory fitness is an important factor in maintaining a healthy body. We know that more people die or are disabled in the Western world by heart attacks (myocardial infarction) caused by cardiovascular disease than by any other medical cause. In elementary terms, cardiovascular disease or coronary artery disease affects the arteries surrounding the heart, eventually clogging them and curtailing the blood supply to the heart. When no oxygen gets to the heart, it dies.

What causes arteries to clog? Usually this is due to arteriosclerosis. The walls of the blood vessels become infiltrated with a fatty plaque which can occlude or block the artery. This doesn't have to happen. Certain factors predispose a person to arteriosclerosis. We know statistically that the rate of this disease is higher when certain factors are present. High blood pressure, diabetes, poor diet, smoking, stress and lack of exercise can all lead to arteriosclerosis. High cholesterol and fat levels in the blood are also shown to be factors.

Many studies have shown that proper nutrition and exercise can help. Under a well-defined fitness program, proper nutrition and exercise can help decrease cholesterol levels, decreasing the incidence of this deadly heart disease. Studies show that the rate of heart attack declines in individuals who exercise on a regular basis, and stress levels have been significantly reduced with regular exercise as well.

**smoking** *(smok-ing) v.t.* **1.** to inhale harmful substances. **2.** to shorten your life. **3.** to cause to be unhealthy. **4.** an incredibly dumb thing to do.

It goes without saying that smoking is self-defeating. Smoking is a major factor in heart disease and lung disease. It shortens the length and reduces the quality of life. If you wish to live a long and healthy life and enjoy cardiovascular respiratory fitness, **don't smoke**!

## THE EFFECT OF FITNESS ON THE MUSCULOSKELETAL SYSTEM

We cannot discuss cardiovascular respiratory fitness without discussing musculoskeletal fitness. The two go hand-in-hand. What good does it do to get your heart rate up to, say, 70% of maximum for 20 minutes at a time, if you end up with a pulled muscle or a stress fracture that keeps you from exercising for the next several weeks? The goal is to be healthy and injury free and, to accomplish both, cardiovascular respiratory fitness <u>and</u> musculoskeletal fitness are needed.

Many different parameters could be used to define fitness of the musculoskeletal system, including flexibility, coordination, strength, postural coordination and overall health of the bone, muscle and soft tissue. As a general definition, *musculoskeletal fitness* is the ability of the body to move to a desired level of exercise without injury. The more fit you are, the less likely you are to sustain an injury.

The musculoskeletal system upon which the movement of the body depends is composed of bones and their associated soft tissue: ligaments, tendons, muscles, fascia, nerves and blood vessels. Exercise can influence development of each of these.

We've talked about some of the changes that occur to muscles with exercise, such as muscle fiber *hypertrophy* (enlargement) or greater muscle mass. There is also an increase in the number of capillaries nourishing the muscle and surrounding connective tissue. As the blood flow improves and proper stress is applied, the connective tissue (fascia, tendons, ligaments and cartilage) will also *hypertrophy* (become thicker), but at a slower rate than the muscle tissue. **The metabolism or**

**aerobic fitness improves first. Next, the muscles get stronger, then the connective tissue and bone.**

Other factors, such as age, are important also. The amount of influence exercise has on the development of the musculoskeletal system depends on individual characteristics as well as the type of training you have chosen.

The development of bone depends on the amount of load applied to the bone. In other words, bone develops stronger in areas that have more load applied. An inappropriate load or too much load, however, can damage the bone, as with stress fractures. Appropriate loads over a long period of time, on the other hand, cause an increase in bone strength along the lines of stress and lowers the likelihood of injury. We know that total inactivity of the bone results in bone absorption and weakness. This is true for ligaments, muscles and cartilage as well.

*Cartilage* is the articular covering on the ends of the bone, lubricated and nourished by the fluids secreted in the synovial membrane. Physical activity keeps the cartilage well nourished. Inactivity makes it soft and easily damaged. Inappropriate stress across the cartilage can damage it. The best method of keeping cartilage in good condition is gentle, appropriate exercise. Unbalanced, extreme loads should be avoided.

*Connective tissue* connects and holds the body together. *Ligaments* and thick connective tissue surrounding the joint (*joint capsules*) work together to hold joints together. *Tendons* connect muscles to bones. *Fascia* is the "packing material" or webbing that surrounds and protects and holds muscles together. Ligaments, tendons, muscles and fascia are formed by connective collagen fibers.

Regular exercise preserves and increases the strength of the connective tissue, the joint capsule, the ligaments and the tendons. Inactivity, however, will cause decrease in strength. It is important in training to realize that the connective tissue and the skeleton and cartilage increase in strength at a slower rate than the muscles. **Just because your muscles are strong does not mean that the connective tissue is ready to handle a heavier load.** Muscles, with exercise, increase in size and strength. Inactivity affects muscles by decreasing their strength, their endurance and their coordination, increasing the risk of injury. Since the healthy, active muscle structure protects the joints and bones from injury by reducing the stress load imposed by impact, it is easy to understand the importance of keeping your muscles in fit condition. The training of the musculoskeletal system includes muscle strengthening, flexibility training, coordination training and *sports-specific training* (performing those exercises which simulate the chosen sport as closely as possible).

## WHAT IS COORDINATION?

Coordination is working the right muscle at the right time efficiently. Most of the time we think of coordination as hand-eye coordination, i.e., perfectly shooting a basket. That is part of coordination, but coordination is also postural coordination or balance coordination. This can also be improved with proper training. With postural coordination and postural strengthening exercises, the muscles tend to become stronger and are available to react when called upon. With postural coordination training, the nerve impulses improve, thus reaction is improved. **Practice improves coordination.**

*Coordination* is the cooperative interaction between the skeletal muscle and the nervous system. *Postural coordination* is the efficient interaction between the skeletal muscles and nervous system to maintain balance. Development of efficient coordination gives improvement in the following areas:

1. Quality of performance.
2. Appropriate responses to balance control with rapidly changing body positions.
3. Grace and beauty of movement.
4. Protection against injuries attributable to awkward movement (*coordination failure injuries—See Chapter Six, Defining Athletic Injuries.*)
5. Efficiency of movement, decreasing chronic overloading of cartilage, bones and other connective tissue (*stress injury—See Chapter Six, Defining Athletic Injuries.*)

## POSTURAL STRENGTH AND COORDINATION

Postural strength and coordination are usually the most neglected part of injury prevention. Even experienced athletes are injured because they have poor postural coordination, even though they are otherwise well-conditioned. Postural coordination is a combination of agility, balance and timing that allows skillful execution of movement. This reduces the risk of injury and heightens the enjoyment of the sport. It is developed by using a great variety of sport-specific agility exercises and drills —also by specific postural coordination and strengthening exercises.

*Strength* refers to amount of force a muscle can generate with muscle *contraction.* In order to increase strength and power of a specific muscle, it must be progressively and gradually challenged or placed under additional stress. This results in hypertrophy (enlargement) of the muscle.

The key here is contraction. A muscle creates no force if it does not contract. To contract, it must receive a nerve impulse. **You can't strengthen what you can't recruit.** *Coordination* is the cooperative interaction between the skeletal muscles and the nervous system. Therefore, coordination must be achieved before strengthening a specific muscle or muscles. In other words, **make the right movements first, then strengthen them.**

Postural strength and coordination refer not just to spinal posture, but also to how the whole body is carried, including the arms and especially the legs. The muscular strength should be sufficient to hold the skeletal structure in good alignment during the shock and strain of exercise. If postural strength fails, the joints will move too far out of their normal range of motion (ROM), unduly stretching the tendinous or ligamentous structures, and injury will occur.

Postural strength should be developed with a series of supplemental exercises emphasizing the development of the muscles of the abdomen, waist, lower and mid back, buttocks, thighs, shoulder carriage and neck. (*See Chapter Four, Individual Training Program for Stretching/Strengthening exercise sets.*)

# STRENGTH TRAINING

The overload principal. In order to cause a physiological response in the muscle that will cause the muscle to hypertrophy (get stronger), resistance must be encountered by the contracting muscle greater than what is normally encountered by that muscle (overload). This must be done gradually and sensibly on a regular basis to achieve significant strength.

As strength increases, the amount of resistance will also need to increase in order to continue to experience overload and continue to gain in strength. Hypertrophy of the muscles is due to increase in size in the individual fibers, not to the increase in the number of muscle fibers. In order to develop strength, it is necessary to work at maximum resistance to get maximum gain. There are three types of exercise: isometric, isotonic and isokinetic.

*Isometric Exercise.* This is a static exercise performed with no motion. It is done with maximum resistance for a short period of time. There is little or no shortening of the muscle during this kind of contraction.

*Isotonic Exercise.* The muscle contracts against the workload and the muscle shortens as the load moves. Push-ups or lifting free weights are examples of isotonic exercise. There are variations in this type of exercise. *Concentric contraction* is contraction with muscle shortening. *Eccentric contraction* is contraction with muscle lengthening.

*Isokinetic Exercise.* This exercise involves constant resistance through a full range of motion. The speed of the motion is also controlled through the entire exercise. A Cybex or Orthotron machine is an example of this.

*Muscle endurance* refers to the muscle's ability to contract repeatedly. Muscle endurance is improved by repetitive movement with small weights. In other words, high repetition of less intensity.

Development of a weight training program. First determine your maximum weight. That is the amount of weight you can lift one to six times comfortably. Using maximum weight, do three sets. Begin by doing four repetitions. Then do six repetitions. In the last set do eight to ten repetitions. If you can do ten repetitions on the third set you should be going to a heavier weight. You should rest four to five minutes between sets. Remember to start out slowly—there is no need to strain or hurt yourself. Gradually increase the weight while allowing your body to adjust. And always, but always, support your lower back.

## SPEED AND ENDURANCE

Muscles are composed of two types of fibers: slow twitch fibers and fast twitch fibers. While the ratio of these is determined genetically, you can make the most of what you have by the type of training you do.

The *slow twitch fibers* are for endurance while the *fast twitch fibers* are for speed and strength. These fibers are quite different from each other—not only in purpose but in physical appearance. Under a microscope, the slow twitch fibers appear red because they are rich in blood supply while the fast twitch fibers appear white because their blood supply is limited. We all have both types and again, that ratio is determined genetically. Great sprinters seem to have a greater percentage of the fast twitch fibers whereas endurance athletes have a greater percentage of the slow twitch variety.

So what does all of this mean to us Everyday Athletes? Not only does it help us to understand our bodies a little better, this information also assists us in deciding **how** we should train. If you want to be a sprinter even though you are basically a slow twitch person, start working on sprints. You may not develop to Olympic class level, but you will develop your fast twitch fibers and improve your sprinting.

This does not mean that you'll gain more fibers. That's not what happens with muscles. <u>You don't gain more fibers; you build and develop the ones you have.</u> That's what body builders do. They don't gain more muscle fibers by weight training, instead, they develop and enlarge the muscle fibers that are already there.

Basically, if you want to improve speed, work on speed. Training fast is important to increasing speed. If you want to improve endurance, work on endurance. And of course, if you wish, you can certainly work on both.

## FLEXIBILITY – STRETCHING

Tight, rigid bodies are more susceptible to injury. Therefore, flexibility is important for injury prevention. Flexibility is also important in comfort and relaxation during heavy exercise, muscular speed and smooth, fluid movement. Conventionally, stretching exercises have been too heavily relied upon for warm-up prior to exercise. When used alone they do not provide an adequately thorough warm-up. They are important as part of the warming-up process, but more important during the cool-down phase.

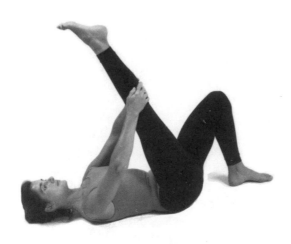

*This shows a position for a hamstring stretch.*

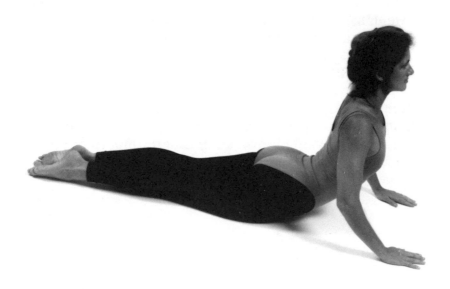

*This shows good flexibility in the lower back area. (See Chapter Four, Individual Training Program, for stretching exercise exact description.)*

The phrase, "No pain, no gain," is misleading when referring to exercises and stretching. When stretching, there should be no severe pain. If your body senses sharp pain as you extend your muscles, chances are you are causing damage to the muscle and perhaps to the ligaments as well. Inappropriate or too much stretching without strengthening or coordination work can be just as bad as too little stretching.

There is a method of exercise that allows for proper stretching and, if carefully adhered to, may even reduce the possibility of injury during a particular sport. (*See Chapter Four, Individual Training Program.*) To sum up, stretching is necessary as part of the warm-up routine, but it must be done correctly.

Flexibility is best developed with a series of stretching exercises emphasizing the Achilles tendon, calf, back of the thigh, knee flexion, hip joint and spinal column. Faster and greater flexibility gains will be achieved when stretching is practiced after exercising. The development of flexibility requires daily practice of stretching exercises until flexibility goals are achieved. Then it should be done regularly as a part of the warm-up and cool-down, to maintain flexibility. No one should neglect regular stretching. Even world class athletes maintain flexibility with a regular stretching program.

## SPORTS-SPECIFIC TRAINING

While working toward achievement in a specific sport (i.e., skiing), try to simulate the sport as much as possible while working out. Work on improving the coordination of the sport, repetitively doing the specific sport over and over again. Improve your speed by exercising at the same speed or faster than in competition. Improve strength by working against resistance in the same manner, working the same muscles that are used in that sport. Sport-specific training works. With it, your body has been trained in the patterns desired, strengthening and conditioning the muscles to be used in the chosen sport. It sure makes the first few days on the slopes a lot more fun and a lot less painful...which leads us to Training and Conditioning. But then, that's another chapter altogether.

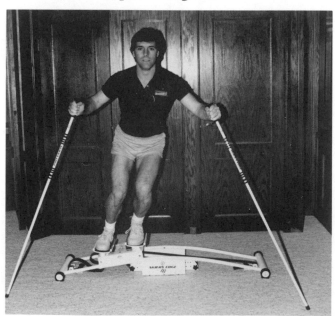

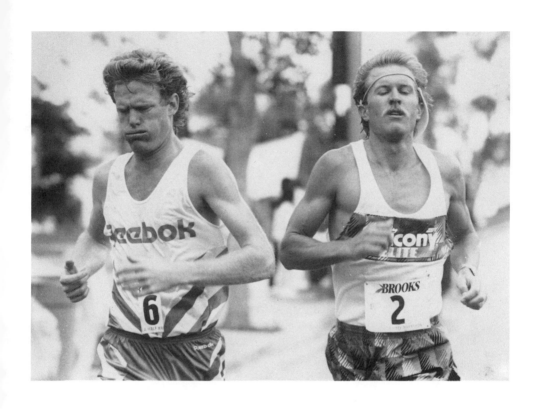

### Chapter Three
# Training and Conditioning

# Training and Conditioning

Okay, Sports Medicine fans, here's the ten-point-toss-up:

Q. Now that you understand what happens to your body
   when you start to train and get fit, "What Time Is It?"
A. Give up? Well, it's time to take a few deep breaths
   and maybe sneak in a few pre-chapter situps and
   pushups. It's time you were formally introduced to
   two brand new friends. Their names are Training and
   Conditioning, and if things go well...they'll be your
   friends for life.

## TRAINING AND CONDITIONING

Regardless of what form of exercise or training program
you choose, or whether you are a beginning or advanced athlete,
every workout should consist of three essential parts:
1. Warm-up, 2. Conditioning and 3. Cool-down.

## WARM-UP PHASE OF EXERCISE

The warm-up prepares the body for the forthcoming exercise. The name of the game is to prevent injuries, and warming-up by doing only stretching just won't do it. There are several changes in the physiological state of the body that need to occur just prior to exercise in order to prevent injury. A good warm-up program accomplishes the following goals:

1. **Increased oxygenation of the blood.** This is provided by increasing the breathing rate, deep breathing and increasing the blood flow to the lungs.

2. **Increased cardiac output.** This is accomplished by mild exercises that increase heart rate gradually.

3. **Increased blood supply to local tissue.** The working muscles, tendons and ligaments should be flooded with blood by warm-up exercises that cause the capillary beds (the smallest blood vessels) to dilate. This increases the temperature. A cold muscle is vulnerable to injury.

4. **Stimulation of points of attachment.** Most injuries are not to muscles but to the sites of muscle attachments—the tendon insertion into the bone. Failure to stimulate and warm-up these points of attachment is probably the most common cause of injury.

5. **Changes in blood chemistry.** A body engaged in moderate-to-heavy exercise requires the blood chemistry to be different than when the body is at rest. Blood quality needs an increase in hormonal secretions (i.e., adrenalin).

6. **Increased synovial fluid secretions.** As the joints warm up, the lubricating fluid secreted by the lining of the joints increases.

7. **Relaxation.** The muscles, tendons and ligaments tend to be relaxed with slow, gentle stretching exercises.

8. **Sport-specific warm-ups.** Slowly and gently go through the basic movement patterns of the upcoming sport, using the equipment, to prepare specific muscles for the vigorous activity required in the conditioning phase. This will also activate the neuromuscular and hand-eye coordination mechanisms.

9. **Psychological preparation.** Mental preparation is important. Think about the forthcoming sports activity. What does it require? Think about it positively. If you are to undergo a difficult or new movement pattern, try to picture it in your mind before doing it. Experience the movement mentally before the warm-up. This is called "*imaging.*" Maybe you have seen world class skiers "*imaging*" at the top of the slope just prior to racing in a downhill World Cup race.

During the warm-up phase and in the slow, cool-down phase, the <u>quality</u> of movement is very important. Concentrate on the pattern of movement even when warming up. Avoid developing bad patterns of movement which will be carried through and reinforced during the conditioning phase if you are not properly using the muscles during the warm-up phase. Practice coordination (using the right muscles) slowly and precisely. This pattern of motion will then be carried through during the conditioning phase. You don't want to strengthen an inappropriate movement pattern. This leads to injury.

These basic principles do not change, although the actual type of warm-up exercises vary somewhat according to the actual exercise to be performed in the conditioning part of the exercise session.

## CONDITIONING PHASE OF EXERCISE

Training usually requires regular increase in activity, causing a **gradually** increased stress to the components involved. The body's tissue response to gradual increases in stress is to build stronger components that help prevent injuries. This is called the *overload principle.*

## PRINCIPLES OF CONDITIONING

**Cardiovascular endurance**. Cardiovascular endurance is best improved by training with the right balance of intensity, duration and frequency. *Intensity* is the pace at which you exercise, *duration* is the number of minutes you exercise, and *frequency* is the number of times per week you exercise.

*The right intensity* is determined by monitoring your training pulse. When you finish your cardiovascular exercise, immediately take your pulse. Beginner's rate should be between 120 and 130 beats per minute, or lower if you are comfortable with that pace. After training at this level for three to six weeks, move up to the intermediate level, which should be 130-140 beats. Conditioned athletes should train at 160 or higher. If your training pulse is too high, you should slow down the pace.

Another way to determine your intensity is to know your *target heart rate*. This is 220 minus your age, times 70%. If you maintain your target heart rate for the right duration, you will achieve the appropriate training effect.

*Duration*: The right duration is determined by monitoring your recovery pulse rate. When you finish your heavy, cardiovascular workout, wait two minutes and take your pulse. Your pulse should have dropped at least 25 to 30%. For example, if you have a training pulse rate of 130 beats per minute, your recovery pulse rate should be 97, two minutes after you finish exercising. If it doesn't recover this quickly, your duration was too long.

*Frequency:* Years ago, competitive runners ran only on weekends and for the total distance they would be racing. Then they discovered that if they ran every day at shorter distances, their racing times improved with less effort and with fewer injuries. After a few decades, they noticed that if they ran every other day and completely rested on the alternate days, they could run even farther and faster during races, with much less weekly training.

The next major breakthrough came when they began to do some very light training on their days off, instead of doing nothing at all. That way they were able to reduce the recovery time and soreness from the heavy training days. Modern research in the physiology of exercise has proven and further refined this *heavy day-light day* concept, along with heavy week and light week patterns that make training safer, more effective and more practical for the Everyday Athlete.

*The right frequency* is a combination of heavy exercise and lighter exercise. Three times a week, every other day, you should exercise at your highest training pulse rate as explained above. On the other two or three in-between days, the intensity should be the same or somewhat easier and the duration should be one third to one half of the heavy days. The easier pace and distance on the lighter days helps your body to clean out the work waste products produced in the tissues on the previous heavy training day. This speeds recovery, prevents soreness and prepares the tissues for the next day's heavy exercise. This five-to-six-day-a-week schedule is the most effective. Every athlete, whether a neighborhood jogger or a world class competitor, should take one day a week off of the regular training schedule to rest.

## COOL-DOWN PHASE OF EXERCISE

Mild exercise, like walking or stretching, after heavy exercise helps to massage the waste products, i.e., lactic acid, out of the muscles. This reduces the time required for recovery from heavy exercise, reduces soreness the next day or two and prepares the tissues for the next day's exercise. This cool-down period should be about the same length as the warm-up routine. During this phase, you adjust to the decrease in the physiological demands slowly rather than abruptly. Specific stretching exercises are done during the cool-down period.

## TRAINING STYLES DURING CONDITIONING

### Aerobic Training

This is by far the most important style of training, whether your purpose is to improve your general health or your athletic performance. Daily runs or walks at a comfortable, steady pace over increasingly longer distances (to a point) have the most positive effect on your health, and lay the foundation for other styles of training and even for competitive running.

*Aerobic training* improves the health of the internal organs in general, and the efficiency of the cardiovascular system specifically. It strengthens the heart and blood vessels, makes the capillary beds more responsive and improves muscular respiration. This means that oxygen and nutrients are delivered to the working muscles more efficiently and work waste products are carried away from the muscles more quickly. You can exercise, work, or play with greater ease. You can enjoy life more and be more productive with less effort.

Consistent aerobic training, together with The Supplementary Exercises, also provides the safe strengthening of the tendon and ligament structures and prevents many injuries that runners are prone to. You should lay a solid foundation with this style of training for at least the first several months before beginning more advanced training styles such as interval training and fartlek.

### Interval Training

*Interval training* is a way of mixing your usual aerobic pace with several repetitions of faster running. For the competitive runner, interval training is a high-intensity form of training that develops speed and strength and cardiovascular endurance to higher levels. It gives more "snap" to leg muscles and sharpens your skill at judging race pace. These intervals should not be sprints, but only slightly faster than the pace you'll be using during a race. You should run at a slower pace for a few minutes in between the faster segments to rest. Interval training for competitive running is both an art and a science in itself.

If you're not a racer but are exercising for general health, you can still use this training style with good effect. First, lay a foundation of aerobic training for several months, until you are running for at least 30 minutes, three times per week. Insert three or four intervals of slightly increased pace into the middle of your normal run. Start by picking up the pace for 20 or 30 seconds and then returning to your usual pace for at least two minutes to rest, then pick it up again, and so on. Gradually increase the length and perhaps the number of the faster intervals.

**Fartlek Training**

Competitive runners have used this training style since it was imported from Sweden a few decades ago. *Fartlek* means "speed play" and it's a free-form kind of interval training. It is perhaps the ultimate for people who run for health. You use your comfortable aerobic pace as a base, and then vary the pace as you feel like it with no prearranged pattern. Speed up, slow down, sprint for a few seconds, jog a little, run sideways or whatever. Just have fun with it!

The beginner needs the safety of carefully constructed, prearranged amounts of running. But <u>after the foundation of conditioning has been laid</u>, fartlek training allows you to break the mold of prearranged paces, distances and times and brings running back full circle to where it belongs. *Play. Fun.* Fartlek training will strengthen you in ways that straight aerobic running can't, but be careful! It's easy to get carried away and overdo.

## MAINTENANCE

Once you reach your goal, you must stay on a regular exercise program in order to maintain that level of fitness. Although the amount of duration, frequency and type of exercise varies with each individual exercise program, certain principles are common to all. You must train three to five days per week for 20 to 30 minutes, with your heart rate at 70% of maximum during training in order to maintain cardiovascular fitness. Cessation of training for two weeks or more causes a significant reduction in training effect. This is true for both the musculoskeletal fitness and for cardiovascular fitness. **Fifty percent of cardiovascular fitness is lost after three months of no training.** Somewhere between two and eight months after cessation of training, the body will revert to its pre-training level of fitness.

## SECOND WIND

After 15 to 30 minutes of cardiovascular exercise (it varies according to your conditioning), you'll experience what is sometimes called a "*second wind.*" It's called that because your breathing will suddenly feel easier, and you'll feel as if your endurance has improved. **It has—but only temporarily.** What's really happened is that your blood chemistry has changed. Your body has adapted to the exercise and your blood is suddenly able to carry oxygen to the working muscles more efficiently. You'll feel lighter, breathe easier, as if you could run a lot longer and a lot farther than you had planned. <u>But don't!</u> Your blood chemistry is temporarily improved, but the condition of your tendons, ligaments and muscles may not be ready for the increase and you could cause an injury. **Be patient and stay with your training plan.**

By the way, this beneficial improvement in blood chemistry lasts for several hours, and that's good for your health. It takes a few minutes to several hours after an exercise session for your blood chemistry to return to "normal," and in the meantime all your cells and tissues are getting the extra benefit.

## OVERTRAINING

Athletes who are successful in their sport and continue to build strength and endurance seem to feel that there is no ceiling to their training and conditioning. This is not so. The body reaches a stage where further training is considered *overtraining*. **Overtraining can be not only harmful, but self defeating as well.** When an athlete overtrains, there is a good chance of experiencing internal fatique that can lead to sports injuries, especially stress-related injuries. Furthermore, continued overtraining leads to retarded progress. This could be labeled "athletic burn-out." Overtraining leaves the player constantly weary and, in turn, this weariness may negatively effect performance. Being constantly tired and not being able to match past performance or experience performance improvement can even lead to depression. This does not need to happen. There is a solution.

**Avoid overtraining.** Do not train hard. Instead, train smart. Allow your body the time for proper fitness and conditioning and always, but always, listen to what your body is telling you. If you are experiencing pain, pull back, evaluate and correct any errors in performance before these errors become injuries. Take advantage of warming up and proper stretching and, finally, ask your body to do only what it has been trained to do. Smart training leads to fewer injuries, much better performance and a happier and more consistent athlete.

## REST – THE OTHER HALF OF EXERCISE

The opposite of exercise is *rest*. It's very important for health and athletic performance to be sure that you get enough rest. This means much more than just getting enough sleep.

Training smart means purposely designing "strategic rest" into your training schedule. That's why light training days should follow heavy ones. One day a week really should be a complete day off from training. Every third week, it's a good idea to reduce the intensity of your workouts a little, then continue increasing the fourth week. Every three months, take a whole week off from training and rest! "Strategic rest" will make you noticeably stronger.

So you see, there's really no mystery to it. Proper Training and Conditioning are yours for the asking. Do your warm-ups, gradually increase your endurance and top off your exercise program with a complete and relaxing cool-down. Stay with your program and reap the benefits that can only be given by Training and Conditioning—those wonderful life-long friends.

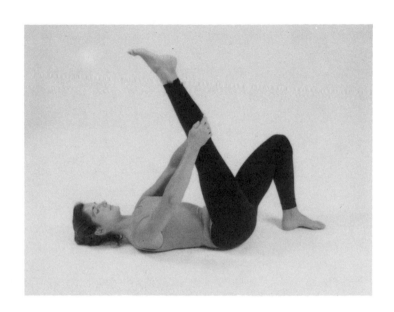

# Individual Training Program

Chapter Four
# Individual Training Program

In selecting a training program of your own, first identify your purpose for training. <u>What are your goals</u>? Do you want the improved health associated with cardiovascular respiratory effects of prolonged exercise? Do you want the "looking good" effects of a fit musculoskeletal system (a "tight bod")? Or do you want a decrease in body injury–the pain-free movement associated with a flexible, strong, well-coordinated body? Do you want the "feeling good" that comes with the psychological and metabolic changes resulting from exercise?

What is your goal? Be realistic. You won't develop a build like Arnold Schwarzenegger without years of training. You won't be able to run a marathon next week, if you've never run before. But given adequate time and a realistic goal you can take a totally inactive, out-of-shape body to a desired level of fitness through a proper training and conditioning program, and then reap the benefits of being fit. Your long-range training program should be planned carefully, taking into account the basic physiological changes that occur so that maximum benefit is achieved and injuries prevented.

In the long-range plan it is important to begin slowly, allowing time (weeks) for the body to build up before challenging it with too much overload. Gradually increase your activity in a well-planned program so that your body builds without injury or setbacks. This could take months or years, depending on your goal. During this building-up phase, you gradually stress the components more and more in order to achieve your goal.

## SUMMARY OF TRAINING PRINCIPLES

### 1. *Cardiovascular Sessions*

All cardiovascular training sessions should include warm-up, conditioning, and cool-down phases. Close attention should be given to the intensity, duration and frequency of the conditioning phase.

A. *Intensity*—This is the *pace* of your exercise. Pick three days of the week for your heaviest training days. On those days, exercise at your target heart rate. The most popular method for obtaining your target heart rate is to subtract your age from 220 and multiply by 70%. On the alternate days exercise at a slightly slower pace.

B. *Duration*—This is the *length* of your exercise session. On heavier training days, exercise for at least 25 to 30 minutes per session at your target heart rate. On lighter training days, cut back to one third or one half the duration of your heavy days.

C. *Frequency*—This is *how often* you exercise. Three heavier days per week, every other day, with three lighter training days in between and one day off each week brings the best results. If you don't feel strong enough on a day that was scheduled as a heavier training day, TRAIN SMART and make that day a light one. If you feel especially strong on the day that was scheduled as a light one, TRAIN SMART and stick to your training plan and train light. Your body still needs the rest.

2. *Supplementary Exercise*

Flexibility, postural coordination and specific postural strengthening exercises should be a part of everyone's program. They can be done following your cardiovascular sessions, or at some other time of the day.

Exercise strengthens muscles but also shortens them and makes them more susceptible to strains and pulls. Also, since tight muscles won't move as far, your stride is shortened with poor flexibility. Stretching lengthens the muscle and relieves tension in the muscle. Light stretching should be done prior to exercise but more thorough stretching should be done after cardiovascular exercise. We'll cover stretching in depth in the *Stretching/Strengthening* Set.

## WARM-UP SET

When practiced consistently, this Warm-up Set makes the ligaments and tendons stronger and yet more pliable and therefore more resilient, dramatically reducing the chance of injury.

An important part of injury prevention is relaxation of the muscles, tendons and ligaments just prior to exercise. To achieve this, do these exercises in a loose fluid manner and avoid any jerky, or tense movements. Try to exaggerate relaxation, and breathe deeply to oxygenate the bloodstream.

Warm-up exercises should be done in a continuous smooth motion with no pauses. Do not force yourself as far into each position as possible, but move only within the comfortable range of motion. Move at a comfortable but brisk pace that makes the pulse rate increase. Start at 10 repetitions of each exercise and build up to 20 repetitions of each. **Also, read the exercises carefully BEFORE attempting them. Note the variations—decide which variations are best for you.** Remember—Take it slow. Allow your body time to get used to anything new.

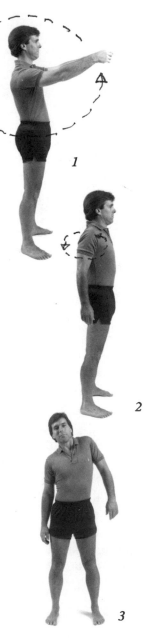

# 1. Arm Circles

**Starting Position** -- *Stand with heels shoulder's width apart and toes pointing slightly to the outside.*

**Execution** -- *Fan the arms in large circles, first in one direction at least 20 times, then reverse (1). Exaggerate the relaxation of the shoulders, arms and hands.*

**Precautions** -- *Be careful for the first few repetitions to be sure that you have no discomfort in the shoulders.*

**Benefits** -- *Relaxes and loosens the entire upper trunk, shoulders and arms.*

**Variation #1: Shoulder Circles** -- *Use this more basic variation just for a change or if the Arm Circles cause discomfort. Keep the arms limp and move the shoulders in the largest circles that you can, 10-20 times, then reverse (2).*

**Variation #2: Single Shoulder Lifts** -- *Raise one shoulder as high as you can. Move the head slightly away from the lifted shoulder so you can raise the shoulder even higher (3). This variation benefits the shoulder area, and also softens chronically tense tissues around the upper thoracic spine.*

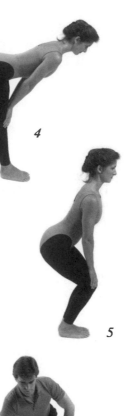

4

## 2. Toes Together Knee Series

**Starting Position** -- *Stand with toes together, hands resting on the thighs just above knees, back straight (4).*

**Execution** -- *1) Bend and straighten the knees, keeping the heels on the floor (4 & 5). 2) Keeping the knees bent, move them from side to side (6). 3) Move knees in large circles, first in one direction, then reverse (7).*

5

**Precautions** -- *Rest the weight of the upper trunk on the hands to avoid straining the lower back. If you have lower back pain during these exercises, move the knees the same way, but carry the back straight up and down. As your back improves from the other exercises, do these exercises with the hands on the knees, but avoid locking the knees during the forward and back exercise (4).*

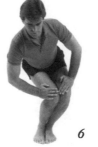

6

**Benefits** -- *Strengthens the ankles, knees, lower thighs and lower back. Makes the ligament structures of the knees and ankles stronger, yet more pliable, thus more resistant to injury.*

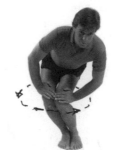

7

## 3. Spinal Flexion/Extension

*Starting Position* -- *Stand with your heels the width of your shoulders apart with the toes pointing slightly to the outside, hands on your hips.*

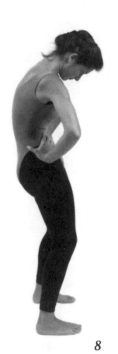

8

*Execution* -- *1) Curl the entire spine forward into a "C" shape. Tuck the tailbone under, tuck the chin to chest. Push the elbows forward to spread the shoulder blades apart, let the shoulders relax. Do not lean the body weight forward (8). 2) Curve the entire spine back in the opposite direction, lower back arched, head back. Pull the elbows back and toward each other to press the shoulder blades together. Do not lean the body weight back (9).*

*Precautions* -- *The forward flexion is safe for nearly everyone, but be careful when extending the neck back and arching the lower back. This is potentially harmful for many kinds of neck and lower back problems. However, move only in a comfortable range of motion, and it should be safe.*

*Benefits* -- *Stretches, loosens and relaxes the tissues of the entire back. Develops suppleness of the spine.*

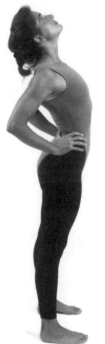

9

*Variation: Neck Forward and Back.* This variation can be used just for variety or when you want to focus on a weak, or habitually tense neck area.

*Execution —* *1)* Tuck your chin toward your chest. Relax the shoulders down *(10)*. Supporting the back of your neck with the fingertips, bend your neck as far back as you comfortably can. Do not open your mouth. Keep your lips together and your teeth touching lightly *(11)*.

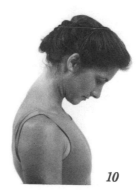

10

*Precautions —* The forward motion is safe for nearly everyone, but be extremely cautious when extending the neck back. If you have a chronically stiff neck, use this exercise and the Neck Rotation (22—see page 46) and Neck Lateral Bend (33—see page 51) in slow motion.

*Caution:* A very popular exercise is to roll the head and neck around in a circle. The front half of this circle is fine as long as you have no particular neck problems, but the back of the circle is a potentially harmful exercise for anyone, and should be avoided. Instead use the Forward and Back, Rotation, and Lateral Bend neck exercises given in this set.

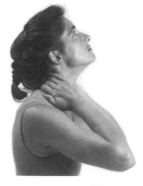

11

## 4. Front Straddle Bounce

*Execution* -- *Bounce up and down. Each time the feet touch down, land with the opposite foot 12-18 inches ahead of the other. Distribute the weight equally on the balls of both feet. Relax the upper body (12 & 13). Build up to 30-60 seconds.*

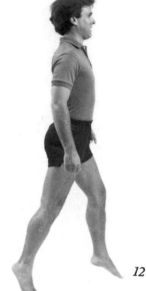

12

*Precautions* -- *Be sure to land very lightly. If you have foot, ankle, knee, back, neck problems, etc., you may have to be careful with this exercise at first, or avoid it altogether until the other exercises strengthen your weak points.*

*Benefits* -- *Strengthens feet, ankles, knees, hips, lower back and spine.*

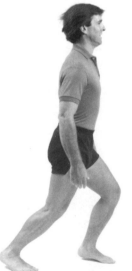

13

## 5. Horizontal Arm Swings, Touch Chest

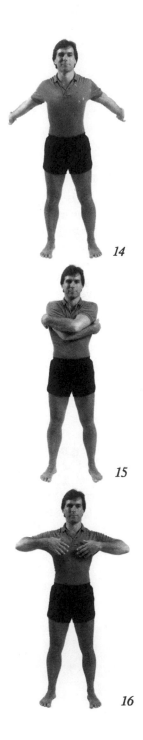

**Starting Position** -- *Stand with your heels the width of your shoulders apart with the toes pointing slightly to the outside.*

**Execution** -- *This exercise is a four-part sequence. 1) Swing your arms back behind you to press your shoulder blades together (14). 2) Swing your arms forward, wrapping them around in front of you as far as you can, letting your arms bounce off your trunk (15). 3) Swing them back behind you again as before (14). 4) Finally, swing them forward again, bending the elbows, and touching the chest (16). This series constitutes one repetition. The entire series should be done at a brisk pace, but in a smooth, continuous motion, like all the warm-up exercises. Exaggerate the relaxation of the shoulders, arms and hands.*

14

**Precautions** -- *Do the first few repetitions cautiously. Be sure to keep your arms below shoulder height. Don't force the swing to the rear.*

15

**Benefits** -- *Relaxes and loosens the whole upper trunk, shoulders, arms and elbows.*

16

## 6. Wide Knee Bends/Legs Straight

*Starting Position* -- Stand with your heels twice the width of your shoulders apart with the toes pointing about 60 degrees to the outside (17).

*Execution* -- 1) Keeping your back upright, bend your knees in the same direction that your toes are pointing. Avoid the tendency to let the knees fall in toward each other by keeping them pulled back so your weight is on the outside edge rather than the inside of the feet (18 & 19). 2) Straighten the legs, fully contract the front thigh muscles; contract the buttocks to flatten the lumbar spine (17).

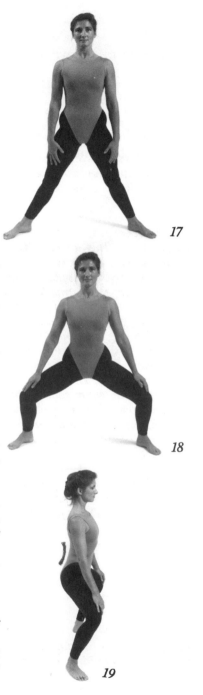

17

18

19

*Precautions* -- Dancers call this Grande Plié, and do it with the lower back flat throughout the exercise. For dance this is correct, but for athletic training, and for weak lower backs, keeping the lower back slightly curved when the knees are bent is safer. If there is any discomfort in the knees, don't completely straighten them, and don't bend as deeply. If you still have knee pain, discontinue this exercise for a time and let the other knee exercises strengthen them.

*Benefits* -- Strengthens the knees, the front of the thighs, the buttocks and the lower back. Helps to retrain the postural strength and coordination between the legs, pelvis and lumbar spine.

# 7. Spinal Twist, Arms Wrap Around

**Starting Position** -- *Stand with the feet shoulder's width apart, with the toes pointing straight ahead.*

**Execution** -- *Keeping the spine erect, twist the entire spine and the hips to the right. Look as far as you can in the same direction (this turns the neck). Swing the arms in the same direction. When twisting to the right, the right hand is in back of the body and bounces off the left waist, the left hand is in front of the body and bounces off the right shoulder. Keep legs straight throughout the exercise. Twist side to side. Completely relax the back, shoulders, arms and hands (20).*

**Precautions** -- *In the beginning it's easy to over-rotate and strain your lower back, so begin each warm-up session cautiously.*

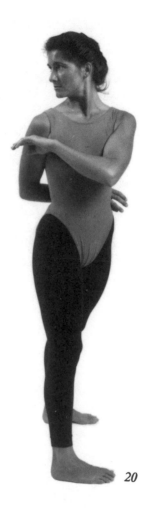

20

**Benefits** -- *Loosens and relaxes the spine, shoulders and arms. Gives the ankles, knees and hips a beneficial twist, difficult to get any other way.*

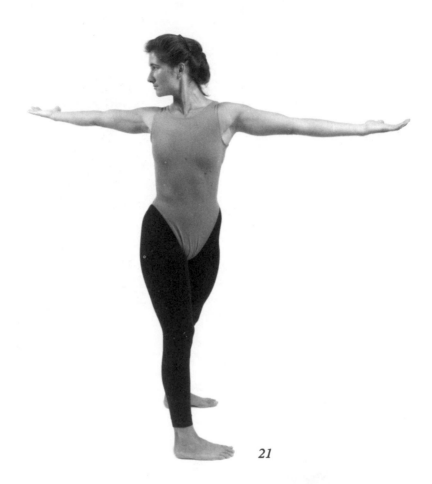

21

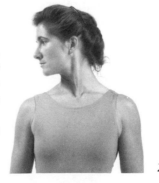

22

***Variation #1: Palms Up Spinal Twist.*** *Use this variation for personal preference or if wrapping the arms around causes discomfort in an injured shoulder. Hold the arms straight out to the sides at shoulder level, palms up, shoulder blades pressing together. Twist to both sides and look at the back hand (21).*

***Variation #2: Neck Rotation.*** *Look as far as you comfortably can to the right (22) and left. Keep the shoulders relaxed down.*

## 8. Side Straddle Bounce

*Execution* -- *Legs do "side straddle hops," but should cross at the ankles. Land with the weight equally distributed on the balls of both feet. Keep the spine erect and the whole body relaxed (23 & 24). Build up to 30-60 seconds.*

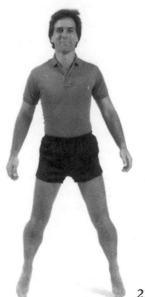

*23*

*Precautions* -- *Be sure to land very lightly. If you have foot, ankle, knee, back, neck problems, etc., you may have to be careful with this exercise at first, or avoid it altogether until the other exercises strengthen your weak points.*

*Benefits* -- *Strengthens feet, ankles, knees, hips, lower back, and spine, and provides the lateral (side to side) strengthening and warm-up that is usually neglected.*

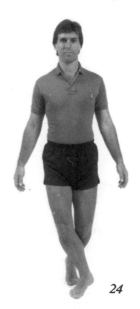

*24*

## 9. Vertical Arm Swings, Touch Shoulders

***Starting Position*** -- *Stand with your heels the width of your shoulders apart with the toes pointing straight ahead.*

***Execution*** -- *This exercise is a four-part sequence. 1) Swing the arms to the front and up above your shoulders as if trying to touch the ceiling and at the same time straighten your ankles and knees (25). 2) Swing the arms down and back behind you with the palms facing to the rear, simultaneously bending the ankles and knees. Lean slightly forward and keep a slight curve in the lower back (26). 3) Keeping the ankles and knees bent, swing the arms to the front and up as before, but bend at the elbows and touch the back of your shoulders (27). 4) Then swing the arms down and back as before, still keeping the knees bent (26). This series constitutes one repetition.*

***Precautions*** -- *Don't lean back when you swing your arms up.*

***Benefits*** -- *Relaxes and loosens the whole upper trunk, shoulders, and elbows. Strengthens the ankles, calves, thighs, lower back and shoulders.*

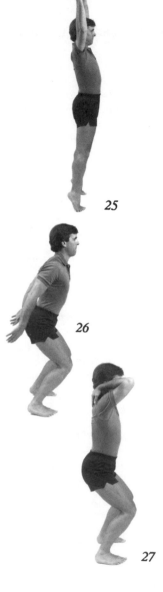

25

26

27

## 10. One Knee Down, Legs Straight

**Starting Position** -- *Take a long step forward, both feet pointing straight ahead and flat on the floor, with 3-4 inches width in your stance, the front of the body facing straight ahead (28).*

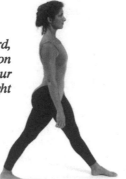

28

**Execution** -- *1) Keeping the back upright, drop the back knee almost to the floor (29). 2) Straighten both legs. Fully contract the front of the thighs and the buttocks (28).*

**Precautions** -- *Avoid leaning forward. The first several days or few weeks, only drop the back knee part way to the floor until you are sure that your knees are strong enough to drop all the way down without strain. If you have any discomfort in your knees, don't go as deep and don't exaggerate the straightening of the knees.*

29

**Benefits** -- *Strengthens the front of the thighs, the knees, buttocks and the lower back. Retrains postural coordination and stability of the legs, pelvis and lower back.*

***Variation: Fencer's Lunge.*** *This is a safer starting exercise if you have pain in the back knee when you do the One Knee Down exercise.*

***Starting Position*** *-- Take a long step forward with the left foot. Point the left foot straight ahead. Point the right foot straight to the right. The heels should line up on a straight line to the front. The front of the body should face to the right. Look straight ahead. Relax the shoulders (30).*

*30*

***Execution*** *-- 1) Bend the front knee straight to the front until its lower leg is vertical. Keep the back knee straight. The forward-most position of the knee should be somewhere above the foot, not beyond the toes. If you want to sink deeper into the final position, but the knee is farther forward than the toes, move the front foot a little forward (31). 2) Straighten both legs (30).*

*31*

***Precautions*** *-- Bending the knee farther forward than the toes may strain the knee. Bend the front knee straight ahead, avoiding the tendency to let it drift to the inside. If you have pain in the front knee, avoid this exercise for a few weeks.*

***Benefits*** *-- Strengthens the ankles, knees, thighs and lower back. Stretches the inner thighs.*

## 11. Spinal Side Bend, Arm Over

*Starting Position* -- *Stand with the feet shoulder's width apart, with the toes pointing straight ahead, and the hands resting low on the hips.*

*Execution* -- *Keeping the legs straight, shift the hips straight to the right and lean the head and shoulders to the left. Lean hard on the left hand to support the upper body weight. This takes strain off the lower back. Relax the neck so that your head drops down as far as comfortably possible. Stretch the right arm over the top (32). Reverse. Move side to side in a smooth continuous motion.*

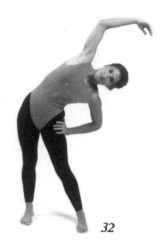

32

*Precautions* -- *Don't try for a full range of motion the first few repetitions of each warm-up session. This direction of movement is very important for the lower back, but has the most likelihood of causing strain if you're not careful.*

*Benefits* -- *Strengthens and relaxes the hip joints, lower back and waist laterally. Stretches the rib cage.*

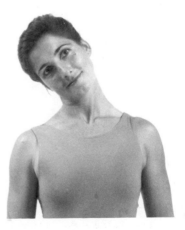

*Variation: Neck Lateral Bend. Use this exercise in a continuous motion for warm-up or slow motion for a weak or sore neck.*

*Execution* -- *Looking straight ahead, relax the head and neck straight to the side as if touching the ear toward the shoulder. Keep the shoulders relaxed down (33).*

33

*Precautions* -- *Use only the comfortable range of motion. You may notice a lot of popping and clicking in the neck at first. These joint sounds are not unsafe as long as there is no pain.*

## 12. Slalom Bounce, Feet Together

**Execution**– *Bounce side to side like a slalom skier. Keep your feet together and your back upright. Land on the balls of your feet. Keep the whole body relaxed (34). Continue for 30-60 seconds.*

34

**Precautions** – *It's easy to slip, so be sure of your footing. Try to land very lightly. If you have foot, ankle, knee, back, neck problems, etc., you may have to be careful with this exercise at first, or avoid it altogether until the other exercises strengthen your weak points.*

**Benefits** – *Strengthens feet, ankles, knees, hips, lower back, and spine, and provides the lateral warm-up and strengthening that is usually neglected.*

## STRETCHING/STRENGTHENING SET
### (Cool Down Phase)

### Slow Motion vs. Fast Motion

There are two kinds of exercises in this set: those for strengthening and those for stretching. Unlike the Warm-up Set, these exercises should be done in slow motion.

When doing the strength exercises, push-ups or sit-ups for instance, slow motion provides muscular development throughout the full range of motion. Doing them faster can leave some portions of the motion weaker.

Entering into the stretching exercises in slow motion is safer and allows the involved tissues to relax more. **Avoid bouncing in the stretched positions.** The bouncing type stretch is called *ballistic* stretching and causes micro tears in the muscle fibers that heal as scar tissue. Holding the stretch instead of bouncing is called *static* stretching and is completely safe provided that the stretch is not entered too far or held for too long. Holding a stretch allows the muscles, tendons and ligaments to adjust to the stretched position gradually, so the muscles don't tighten defensively.

**Don't force too far into the stretches.** You should feel a good stretch, but never pain. If you try to force it you will retard your progress and may cause soreness. You may even cause strains or sprains that will keep you from exercising and may require medical care. Let your body's comfort level determine how far to enter the stretches and how long to hold them. **Always be comfortable.**

Each repetition of a strength or stretching exercise should take 6 seconds to execute, then pause for 2 seconds in the final position. Then move in the opposite direction on a 6 second count and pause again for 2 seconds in that final position. Move for 6, pause for 2. Do only 6-10 repetitions of each exercise.

The pauses in the final stretching positions should be kept at 2 seconds in the beginning. After the first 2-3 weeks of daily training, if you want to emphasize certain stretches, do only one repetition, but gradually hold the stretch longer, building up to 30-60 seconds, and even longer if you like after another few weeks.

## 1. Calf and Achilles Stretch

**Starting Position** -- *Hands against a wall, post, railing, etc. Take a long step back with one foot. Point the toes of both feet straight ahead.*

35

**Execution** -- *1) Keep the back knee locked straight. Bend the front knee and shift weight forward. This directs the stretch to the upper calf. Hold for 30-60 seconds (35). Stretch the other leg. 2) Next, bend the back knee. This directs the stretch to the lower calf and Achilles tendon. Hold for 30-60 seconds (36). Reverse.*

**Precautions** -- *Lean the upper body slightly forward to avoid over-arching the lower back. Be sure to keep the outside edge of the back foot pointed straight ahead to avoid collapsing the arch of the foot.*

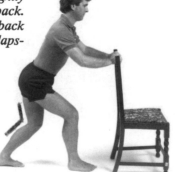

36

**Benefits** -- *Walking, jogging and many other forms of exercise strengthen the calf muscles, which become shorter, tighter and more prone to injury. These two exercises maintain flexibility of the calf and Achilles tendon.*

## 2. Standing Quad Stretch

*Starting Position* -- *Hold on to something for balance. Stand on your left foot. Reach behind you with your left hand and hold the right foot.*

*Execution* -- *Lift the right foot up and to the rear to draw the right knee to the rear (37). Reverse.*

*Precautions* -- *Holding the opposite foot keeps the hips and lower back in a straight alignment. If there is any discomfort in the knee area, don't lift as high. If you still have discomfort, you may have to avoid this technique until your knees are made stronger with the other knee exercises.*

*Benefits* -- *As the front of the thigh (quad-riceps) gets stronger with exercise, it also shortens, which can interfere with the safe, fluid motion of the knee joint, and how you carry the pelvis and lower back. This maintains its flexibility.*

37

## 3. Kneeling Hip Stretch

*Starting Position* -- *Kneel with the right knee on the floor and the left foot flat on the floor. Rest the hands on the left thigh and lean the upper trunk slightly forward.*

*Execution* -- *Step out farther with the left foot and lower the hips to increase the stretch. The left foot should remain flat on the floor and the left lower leg should be vertical. (38). Reverse.*

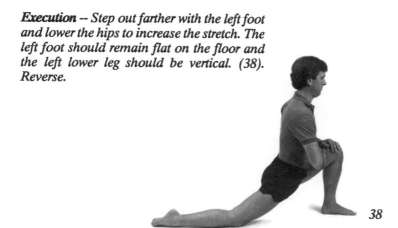

*38*

*Precautions* -- *Avoid leaning the upper body back as this may strain the lower back.*

*Benefits* -- *Maintains flexibility of the hip flexor muscles (iliopsoas group), the front of the thigh (quadriceps), and the hip joint.*

# 4. On All Fours, Spinal Flexion/Extension

***Starting Position*** *-- The quadruped (on all fours) position with the hands directly under the shoulders and knees directly under the hips.*

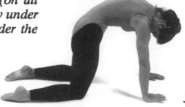

*39*

***Execution*** *-- 1) Flex (curl forward) the entire spinal column, tuck the tailbone under, lift the middle spine up, and tuck the chin toward the chest to fully flex the neck (39). 2) Extend (arch back) the entire spine; <u>gently</u> increase the curvature of the lower back. Try to arch the area between the shoulder blades, and lift the head and neck back carefully (40).*

***Precautions*** *-- Extreme care should be taken when extending (arching back) the lower back and the neck, whether or not there is a history of neck or lower back problems. Most people need to increase the flexibility and strength of the spine, but it must be done cautiously.*

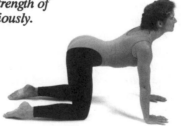

*40*

***Benefits*** *-- Relaxes the musculature of the lower and middle back and the neck. Helps to re-establish the suppleness and stability of the whole spinal column.*

## 5. Toe and Knee Bend

***Starting Position*** -- *Kneeling with the toes bent under (pointing forward), the balls of the feet and the heels touching, the knees a few inches apart (41).*

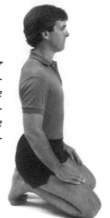

*41*

***Execution*** -- *Slowly sit back on the heels (42), then raise up to the starting position.*

***Precautions*** -- *Keeping the heels together properly aligns the knee joint. If any knee discomfort is experienced, this exercise should be done from a quadruped (on all fours) position and very cautiously. If you still have knee pain, discontinue until the other knee exercises stretch and strengthen the knees.*

*42*

***Benefits*** -- *Re-establishes flexibility of the feet, Achilles tendons and knees; strengthens the lower front of the thighs and ligamentous structure of the knees.*

## 6. Push-ups

***Starting Position*** -- *Push-up position with hands directly under the shoulders; upper legs and trunk in a straight line; look straight at the floor (43).*

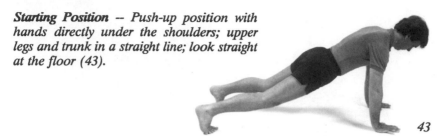

*43*

***Execution*** -- *As you slowly lower to the floor, the thighs, stomach and chest should reach the floor at the same time (44). When you push off the floor they should leave the floor at the same time. Do not let the head and neck sag downward, which often leads to poor head/neck posture. Pull the nose back as far from the floor as possible and look directly at the floor. This keeps the head and neck in proper alignment with the rest of the spine. Keep the shoulders pressed down away from the ears throughout the exercise.*

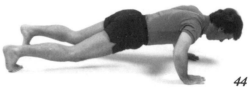

*44*

***Precautions*** -- *If you have neck problems it may be difficult to hold the weight of the head up for the time required for this and some other exercises. Start with fewer repetitions and gradually increase, or sit back on the heels and rest every few repetitions until you get stronger.*

***Benefits*** -- *Strengthens the arms, shoulders and chest and if properly executed, improves the habitual carriage of the shoulders.*

***Variation:*** *If you don't have the strength to do the push-ups using this form, do them from the knees instead of from the balls of the feet and/or don't lower yourself as far.*

## 7. Foot and Ankle Series

*Starting Position* -- *Sit on the floor with the knees bent, heels resting on the floor. Keep the ankles bent at 90 degrees.*

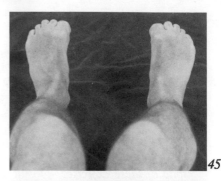

*Execution* -- *1) Curl the toes as far forward as you can. Clench down hard for 2 seconds (45), then curl them back as hard as possible and hold for 2 seconds (46). Repeat 6-10 times. 2) Next, curl the great toes back hard and the other toes forward hard, hold 2 seconds (47), then reverse positions and curl the great toes forward hard and the other toes back hard, hold 2 seconds (48). Repeat 6-10 times. 3) Next, keeping the ankles bent at 90 degrees, pull the ankles to the inside (inversion) hard so that the soles face each other, hold 2 seconds (49), then push the ankles to the outside (eversion) hard as if trying to face the soles to the outside, hold 2 seconds (50). Repeat 6-10 times.*

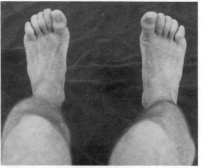

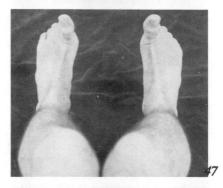

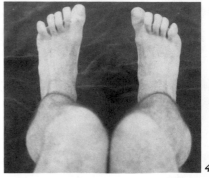

*Precautions* -- The muscles in the feet may cramp at first, but it should pass after the first several days or few weeks. If you have persistent foot or ankle pain or fatigue in spite of these exercises, consult a podiatrist or orthopedist specializing in sports injuries. Cramping or inability to control the toes and feet in these exercises indicates a serious need for strengthening.

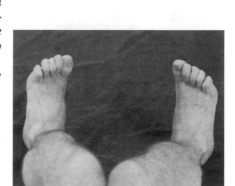

49

*Benefits* -- When we start exercising, the muscles and ligaments in our feet are often so weak from sedentary habits and being confined in shoes so much, they often can't take the stress of exercise. This frequently leads to foot and ankle injuries. Used consistently, these exercises can help to strengthen the involved structures and prevent injury.

50

## 8. Sit-ups

***Starting Position*** -- *Assume a back-lying position with knees raised and the feet flat on the floor, arms resting across the abdomen (51).*

***Execution*** -- *Slowly sit up far enough to raise the shoulder blades off the floor. Hold for 2 seconds (52). Return slowly to the floor and immediately repeat. Continue until the abdominal muscles are fatigued.*

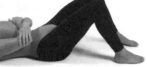

51

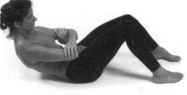

52

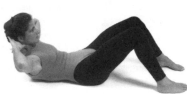

53

***Precautions*** -- *Sitting up higher than is pictured is unnecessary and can lead to low back strain. Do not tuck the chin to the chest. This can produce strain in the back of the neck or upper back. Avoid the opposite mistake of looking at the ceiling which can perpetuate a poor head and neck posture. A convenient guide is to carry the chin "one fist's distance" away from the chest, and look over the top of the knees as you sit up. If you feel discomfort in the sides or back of the neck, support the back of the head with the fingertips (53).*

**Benefits** -- *Strong abdominal muscles are important for strong pelvic and spinal carriage. The abdominal muscles are arranged in four separate layers that run in different directions. The sit-up described above strengthens the muscle fibers that run vertically from the pubic bone to the rib cage. This basic sit-up should be used for a week or more before starting the variations below. The more advanced versions develop the vertical layers and also the oblique layers of the abdominal wall. If no discomfort is felt in the lower back, this side to side method is far safer for the lower back and develops the abdominal area quicker and more thoroughly than the usual kinds of sit-ups.*

**Variation #1:**  *Slowly sit up far enough to raise the shoulder blades off the floor (52). Keeping the shoulder blades off the floor, slowly shift to one side as if looking around the knees, rotating the trunk slightly (54). Pause 2 seconds, then shift to the opposite side. Pause 2 seconds, then slowly shift back to the center, and then lower to the floor. Repeat until abdominals are fully fatigued.*

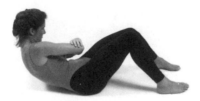

*54*

**Variation #2:**  *Repeatedly shift side to side without returning to the floor. Remember to use slow motion and pause for 2 seconds at the far left and right positions. Continue until fatigued.*

## 9. Back-lying, Hamstring Stretch

*Starting Position* -- *Lie on your back with one knee bent and its foot flat on the floor, the opposite leg straight up with its knee slightly bent, hands on the back of the knee.*

*Execution* -- *Pull the leg back gently until you feel a mild stretch in the back of the thigh (55).*

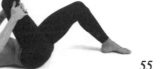

55

*Precautions* -- *Be sure the tailbone stays on the floor. Relax the head and shoulders to the floor. Keeping the leg slightly bent directs the stretch to the back of the thigh only. Stay with this method for at least the first 2-3 weeks before going on to the variation.*

*Benefits* -- *The muscles of the back of the thigh and the tendons that connect them to the bones are often too rigid, or become too short when they are strengthened by regular exercise. This exercise maintains the flexibility of those tissues, which allows freedom of movement and proper carriage of the knee joint, pelvis and lower back.*

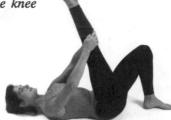

56

*Variation:* *Keeping the leg you're stretching completely straight stretches the hamstrings (back of the thigh), and also the back of the knee and upper calf (56).*

## 10. Back-lying Spinal Twist

**Starting Position** -- *Back-lying with knees pulled up toward chest, hips resting on the floor, arms out to the sides a little lower than shoulder level.*

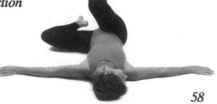

57

**Execution** -- *Relax the legs to the side and down to the floor. In the final position, keep the knees pulled up toward the arm and attempt to keep both shoulder blades on the floor. Rotate the head and neck as far as you comfortably can in the opposite direction (57).*

58

**Precautions** -- *If any strain is felt in the lower back while lowering or raising the knees, lower one leg at a time, then raise one leg at a time (58). If any pain is felt while in the final position, restrict the range of the motion by lowering the legs only part of the way to the floor. Gradually enter farther into the final position as you grow stronger and more flexible.*

**Benefits** -- *Relaxes and improves flexibility of the entire spinal area. Strengthens the lower- and mid-back and the oblique and transverse abdominal layers.*

## 11. Side-lying Quad Stretch

***Starting Position*** *-- Lie on the left side with the head resting on the left arm. Hold the right foot with the right hand.*

***Execution*** *-- Pull the right foot back to stretch the front of the thigh (59).*

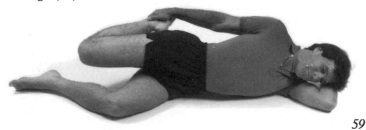

59

***Precautions*** *-- If there is any discomfort in the knee area, don't pull the knee as far to the rear. If you still have discomfort, you may have to avoid this technique until your knees are made stronger with the other knee exercises.*

***Benefits*** *-- This exercise maintains flexibility of the front of the thigh.*

## 12. Front-lying Press-ups

***Starting Position*** *-- Lying face down with the hands under the shoulders like a push-up position, legs together.*

***Execution*** *-- Push up with the arms, arching the lower back, but keep the hips on the floor. Look straight ahead. Keep the shoulders pressed down away from the ears (60).*

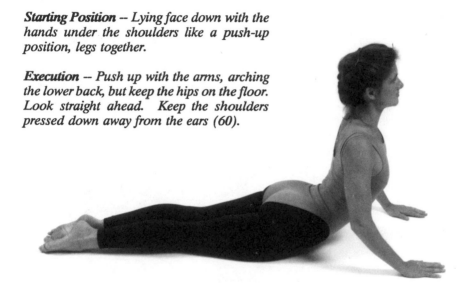

*60*

***Precautions*** *-- This method is inappropriate for a few kinds of back problems, but beneficial for most if done carefully. If you have a history of low back pain, check with a physician who specializes in low back problems before proceeding. Be sure to keep the buttocks tense to protect the lower back from over compression.*

***Benefits*** *-- Helps to normalize lumbar range of motion and strengthens the buttocks and lower back.*

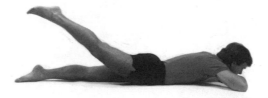

*61*

## 13. Front-lying Leg Lifts

***Starting Position*** *-- Lying face down, chin resting on hands, legs together.*

***Execution*** *-- Slowly lift one leg off the floor as high as you comfortably can, keeping the knee straight.   Pause for 2 seconds, then slowly lower to the floor (61).  Alternate legs. Use this easier variation for 2-3 weeks before advancing to the other variations.*

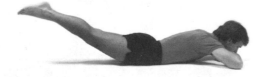

*62*

***Precautions*** *-- If you have any pain in the lower back, don't lift as high. If you still have pain, discontinue this exercise for a time while the other exercises strengthen your back.*

***Benefits*** *-- Strengthens the entire low back area and the buttocks.*

**Variation #1:  *Front-lying Double Leg Lifts***
*Slowly lift both legs off the floor, as high as
you comfortably can and pause for 2 seconds (62). Slowly lower to the floor.*

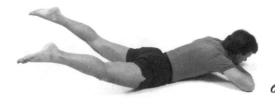

*63*

**Variation #2:  *Legs Open and Close*** *-- Keeping the legs together, slowly lift them off the
floor (62), then spread them apart and pause
for 2 seconds (63). Press them together again
before lowering to the floor.*

## 14. Back-lying Hold Knees

*Starting Position* -- *Back-lying with knees up toward chest, hands holding each other, wrapped around the upper shins, head and hips resting on the floor (64).*

*Execution* -- *Relax the muscles of the shoulders, arms, legs and hips, then the muscles of the lower and mid-back will relax.*

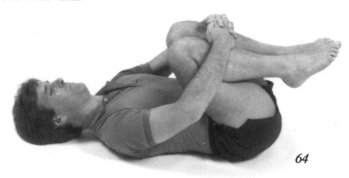

*64*

*Precautions* -- *Don't pull the knees back toward the chest, just relax. If the knees are sensitive to a full bend, put the hands between the calves and the thighs instead. Avoid the tendency to press the back of the head against the floor.*

*Benefits* -- *Loosens the hip joints and the knees. Relaxes the lower and middle spine and gives them a mild traction.*

Although we have described precautions and variations to the exercises to make this a potentially injury free exercise program, checking with your physician or orthopedic surgeon prior to beginning a program is always advisable.

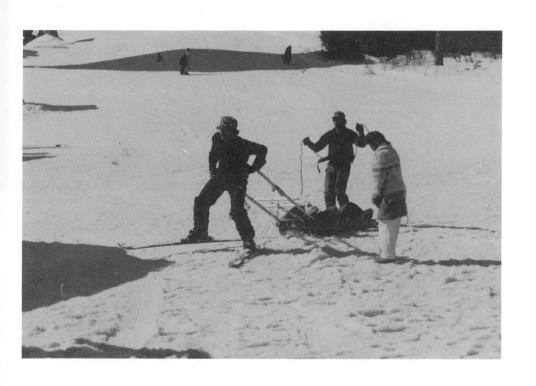

Chapter Five
# Basic Causes of Sports Injuries

## Chapter Five
# Basic Causes of Sports Injuries

**in-jure** *(in'jer)* *v.t.* **-jured 1.** to inflict bodily damage; to miss out on all the fun; to be hobbled; to spectate; to hang out with nothing to do; to be limping rather than playing.

Famous last words of persons voted to be most likcly to get injured:

"I'll make sure to warm up good.... NEXT time."
"Hey...forget about that stuff! Stretching is for wimps."
"My philosophy is to go as hard as I can for as long as I can."
"Gee, my leg is really sore...but I'm sure it'll loosen up as we go."

It is important to understand the three basic causes of sports injuries that occur to the musculoskeletal system. These are injuries due to *direct trauma, coordination failure* and *stress injuries*.

## DIRECT TRAUMA

Jim, an expert skier, left the lift with a swish. His form was excellent. He maneuvered on the slope seemingly without effort. He executed a quick turn at the crest of the second slope and prepared to make a lateral hop at the junction of two runs. Jim decided to round the edge of the slope on the far side, near a grove of pines. Another skier, somewhat out of control, rammed him from the side and sent Jim off course, driving him into a tall pine. Jim's shoulder took the brunt of the impact against a solid tree trunk. He came to an abrupt halt and fell at the edge of the slope in great pain. Within an hour, the Ski Patrol had Jim off the mountain and into a clinic, where an orthopedic surgeon examined him.

> SYMPTOMS....Extreme pain and decreased function, deformity over the collar bone.

> DIAGNOSIS..."Fractured clavicle" or broken collar bone.

Jim's injury was caused by *direct trauma*. He had control, balance and agility, but he was in the wrong spot at the wrong time and suffered a sports-related injury.

*Direct trauma* is an injury caused by hitting a person or an object. In skiing, this could be caused by hitting a tree, a rock, another skier, or standing in a lift line and being hit by another skier. In football, this kind of injury could be caused by ramming into another player, or by that other player hitting you, or by your body hitting the ground. In diving, it may mean hitting the board or bottom of the pool. In ice skating, it might mean hitting the wall or taking a hard fall on the ice. In other words, a sudden collision with any object can cause injury.

This illustration shows a football player being clipped. Clipping can result in a knee injury common to contact sports. This *direct trauma* injury is caused when a player is hit from the side. That contact may result in torn ligaments. Another *direct trauma* injury can result when a player falls and hits the ground hard. Falling and landing on the knee, for example, may result in a dislocation or a fracture of the knee.

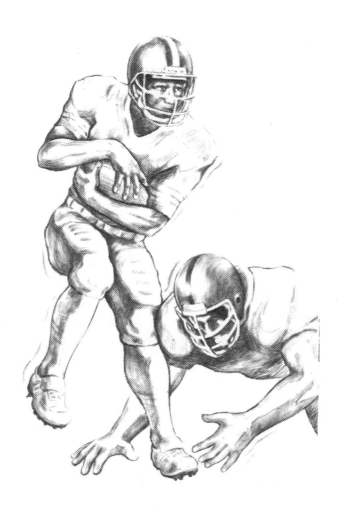

*Football player being clipped, which can result in a knee injury common to contact sports. This is an example of a direct trauma injury, a blind-sided direct hit from another player, causing ligament damage.*

## COORDINATION FAILURE

Sally was the best tennis player Southwestern College had trained in years. Her skill and agility was touted in the local papers. At 18, she had a great future. While in competition one spring afternoon, Sally's opponent returned a surprisingly fast ball to the right court. Sally, quickly reversing direction, forced her lower legs to move in one direction and her thigh and body to zag in the opposite direction. Her instructor heard the ligament pop in Sally's right knee. The knee immediately felt loose, and the tennis star fell to the court in great pain—unable to support her body weight. At an emergency care unit, the following determinations were made:

SYMPTOMS....Severe pain, swelling, looseness of the joint.

DIAGNOSIS....Severe torn ligament in the right knee or a third-degree sprain.

Sally was placed on the sidelines by *coordination failure*. Whenever the body is contorted in a manner that exceeds the limits of the muscular/skeletal ability to adjust properly to drastic movements, something has to give. It may be a shoulder joint, a knee ligament or a muscle. Even the most vibrantly alert player of sports can and sometimes will experience *coordination failure*. When the muscles don't react perfectly, or in harmony, for the attempted movement, it causes an imbalance. No outside force causes the injury; instead, it results from the appropriate muscles failing to work together at the right time.

*Coordination failure* injuries result principally from a momentary loss of balance. This is a common cause of injury, especially to the knee. It is a weight-bearing, twisting injury that may result in a torn ligament (sprain), a tear of the *meniscus* (cartilage in the knee), a *fracture* (broken bone), dislocation of the kneecap (patella) or a combination of all these injuries.

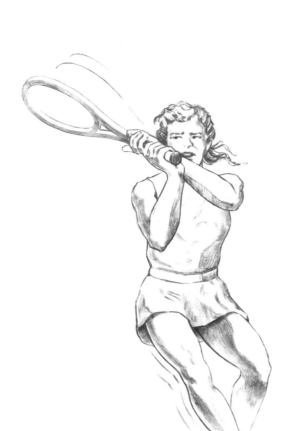

*A coordination failure type injury—the lower leg remains planted
while the upper body rotates, creating undue stress across the
knee ligaments resulting in a ligament tear.*

## STRESS INJURIES

Fred refused to let up. He had finished the Brownfield 10K run every year since he graduated from college. At 29, he prided himself on his fitness. Most of his buddies were beginning to show flab, and he didn't want that to happen to him. But on this particular morning, Fred couldn't finish the race. Just 4K into the run, his legs were in too much pain to continue. He lay in the street in great pain.

The next morning, stiff but able to walk, Fred called his orthopedic surgeon, who asked to see him that day. This was not Fred's first visit to his orthopedic surgeon. As a matter of fact, his doctor had cautioned him about potential problems resulting from stress to his legs. His doctor had even recommended that Fred see a physical therapist to develop a flexibility and coordination program to try to avoid possible stress injuries. Fred had scoffed at the idea. After all, he had been an outstanding athlete throughout his high school and college years. What could a physical therapist possibly do for him?

Finally realizing that something needed to be done, Fred agreed to make an appointment with a physical therapist as his doctor recommended.

SYMPTOMS....Aching pain in the lower leg.

DIAGNOSIS...Overuse of the posterior tibial muscle, causing shin splints.

Fred's story is, unfortunately, not unique to runners. He experienced a very common *stress* or *overuse* injury. Among runners, it's the most common type of injury, usually the result of incorrect or inadequate training. The effect this can have on the body is much like driving a car when it is out of alignment, and the results can be much the same.

A *stress injury* can happen to almost any part of the musculoskeletal system. It is a breakdown of tissues caused by repetitive application of force at a rate exceeding the healing capacity of the tissues. In short, a stress injury is a wearing-out process.

## OVERUSE

Too often, the new as well as the seasoned athlete will ask his or her body to do more than it has been trained to do. This is called "overuse." In the past, too much emphasis has been placed on the term "overuse" and not enough on the actual cause of the injury related to it. Before the upsurge in sports medicine, the solution to any sports injury was to stop the athlete from participation in sports altogether. Now we ask why the injury happened, what is necessary to repair the injury and what can we do to prevent it from happening again?

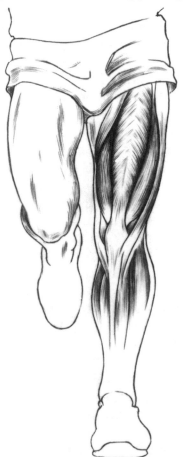

*Stress injury—Running produces approximately four times the stress across the lower legs and the knees as walking.*

Why did the injury occur? Was it lack of proper preparation, flexibility or postural coordination? Was it a result of direct trauma? Perhaps it was a combination of these. A would-be athlete who demonstrates poor flexibility, coordination, strength and endurance, yet tries to run a marathon, will end up getting hurt. Technically, that could fit in the category of overuse. Certainly, it is correct to say that running a marathon was too strenuous for that particular body to handle. The same could be said of a person who has been completely inactive for years who, after donning shorts and shoes, with no warm-up or conditioning, proceeds to run for 30 minutes. He discovers the next morning that he is not only very sore, but has a severe case of shin splints and should not run again until they are healed. This person asked his body to do more than it was trained to do.

Are you in condition to do the sport you have chosen to do? Be honest! Even if you once were a good tennis player, skier, football player or track star, if you have been inactive for several months or years, you are not in condition to jump in and start playing without risking injury. Your mind might be willing but your body lacks the proper preparation.

On the other hand, you may be a very active person—a weekly racquetball player and a seasoned runner. Does this mean that you are in condition to step into your bindings and race down the hill directly following the first major snowfall? Not necessarily. Even though you are an active athlete, you may still need to perform certain strengthening and stretching exercises that are *sport-specific* (simulating the chosen sport as closely as possible) in order to protect your body from being asked to do what it is not trained to do and thus risking unnecessary injury. You may be one of the millions of people who have never been athletic—someone who would like to increase their activity and become a walker, a runner or learn to play tennis. Being in condition first may make the difference between becoming an athlete comfortably and happily or sustaining an injury and quitting altogether.

The correct method of conditioning and proper training is to go at it gradually. **Don't rush yourself into shape.** Go slow and allow your cardiovascular respiratory system to develop. **Give your musculoskeletal system the time and conditioning it needs to sustain the movement necessary without becoming**

**injured.** Be aware of your body's level of training and conditioning and try not to exceed it. If you take the time for proper training and conditioning and approach your chosen sport with a realistic sense of timing, you can become the athlete you want to be and avoid many of the injuries associated with your chosen sport.

There are three basic categories into which injuries can be classified: 1. Direct Trauma, 2. Coordination Failure, and 3. Stress or Overuse. It is not unusual for injuries to result from a combination of these. For example, you've been skiing too many days in a row, and your patellar tendon shows signs of tendinitis (*stress injury*). The pain causes the muscles not to work properly. You go over a bump, the timing of the muscles is off, one leg goes the wrong way (*coordination failure*) and you fall. You hit the ground with your hand outstretched, tearing the ligaments in your thumb (*direct trauma*).

You see, injuries don't always fall into one category or another, but categorizing injuries helps you recognize the ways injuries occur, so you can better prevent them. For instance, if you know what causes stress injuries or overuse injuries, you can prevent them by training properly and exercising intelligently. With proper agility, coordination and sport-specific strength training, many coordination failure injuries can be prevented. Although the injuries from direct trauma can be decreased by training and conditioning (you'll hit the ground less), many injuries due to direct trauma cannot be prevented (you can still be crushed by a 400 lb. "*Refrigerator*"). But the better shape you are in, the easier the treatment course. **There are fewer severe injuries, in general, in people who are in good physical and mental condition than those who are not.**

When discussing injuries, other factors, including weather conditions and equipment are frequently involved. This includes using pads and helmets for collision sports, ski boots and bindings appropriate for your level of skiing, as well as properly fitted running shoes. It is important to know your sport, use suitable equipment and always ask for professional help if needed.

**It is also important to listen to your body and use good sense.** If you feel pain, perhaps that's your body's way of telling you something is wrong. If the pain continues, acknowledge it, and try to understand what your body is saying. Seek to understand your injury, how it is being caused, and what you can do to prevent or heal it. **Then you can become an active member of the Sports Medicine Team—reducing risks and preventing injury.**

**pre-ven-tion** *(pre-ven'shun) n.* **1.** Knowing how it happens; understanding why it happens; learning as much as you can and doing your darnedest so it doesn't happen to you.

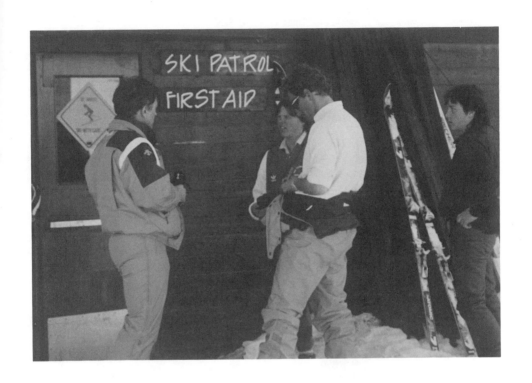

# Defining Athletic Injuries

## Chapter Six
# Defining Athletic Injuries

Okay, Sports Medicine Fans, here's the question. You're shopping at a neighborhood grocery store when you somehow miss the cart with a six-pack of double ply Charmin.[R] Then, to compound the trauma, you run over it with all four wheels. Do you think that constitutes a SOFT TISSUE INJURY?

I sure hope you said, "No!"

### SOFT TISSUE INJURIES

Soft tissue injuries include contusions, hematoma, ligament sprains, strains, bursitis, muscle cramps and soreness. Lacerations, cuts and blisters can also be included in this category. First, what is soft tissue? There are eight soft tissues and, although it's hard to believe, not one of them begins with a C, ends with N and sometimes ends up on the floor of a grocery store underneath a shopping cart. Soft tissue consists of ligaments, tendons, muscles, nerves, blood vessels, fat, fascia and skin.

## CONTUSION

A *contusion* is commonly thought of as a bruise. This is usually caused by a direct blow to the soft tissue. The blow causes damage to the soft tissue resulting in bleeding into the damaged area. Then there is a clotting of the blood which stops the bleeding. The discoloration associated with a contusion is the accumulation of this clotted blood. The severity of the contusion depends on the amount of damage caused by the direct blow, and is usually related to the location and the severity of the tissue damage.

A mild bruise will cause almost no secondary problems. It can be easily treated with icing and the athlete can quickly return to activity. More severe contusions need to be treated immediately with icing, compression and elevation, and sometimes require more involved treatment by the therapist or trainer. In some cases, severe contusions can put an athlete "on the bench," so it is important that these be treated immediately and by a professional.

## THE HIP POINTER

The *hip pointer*, a common sports injury, is a contusion of the muscle that lies over the iliac crest (*See Illustration*). This is the large muscle that forms over the outside of the palpable pelvic bone or hip bone. This muscle is usually injured when it is mashed between the bone and a hard surface such as turf. A "direct blow" type of injury, it is commonly seen in contact sports.

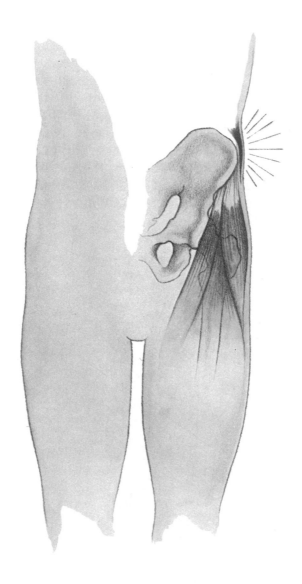

*The hip pointer -- the contusion over the iliac crest.*

## HEMATOMA

A more severe injury which causes a large accumulation of blood in the soft tissue is called a *hematoma*. Accumulated blood clots in the tissue and forms a solid, swollen area. As it heals, the clot is slowly broken down and absorbed by the body. It is important to understand that a hematoma is not the kind of clot that travels to the heart or lungs, such as the condition of clots in blood vessels, called *thrombosis*. Hematomas, instead, are well localized and do not travel, but they can cause secondary problems locally. Because of the size of the hematoma, it usually causes distending (swelling) of the tissue, secondary pain, and limited motion. This can cause a shutdown of the muscles around the hematoma, resulting in flexibility problems or coordination failure.

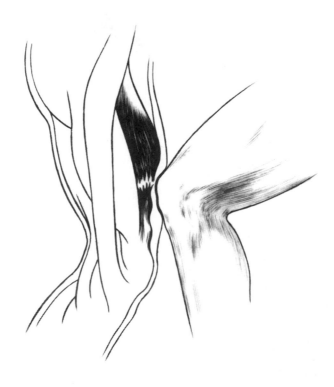

*A contusion to the thigh muscles due to a direct blow.*

A secondary problem with hematoma is that sometimes, instead of being completely absorbed by the body, the blood clot within the muscle will *calcify* (become hard with deposits of calcium). This is called *myositis ossificans*. This condition needs to be seen and treated by a medical specialist to avoid permanent injury to the muscle and to the extremity.

Even a less severe hematoma may cause the shutdown of a particular muscle, leaving the area weaker and more susceptible to a secondary injury. An example would be an injury to the *quadriceps muscle*, which helps to stabilize the knee. With weakened quadriceps, the knee is less likely to be stable, making it more vulnerable to injury. Severe bruises or hematomas should be seen and treated by your health professional.

Sometimes even a mild hematoma can cause a shutdown of a muscle and thus effect a joint. In this instance, the athlete may continue to participate, calling on the injured muscle to perform. **Since it can't, the body will compensate for the one that is shutdown by substituting another.** When this happens, it's like playing cards without a full deck. The athlete is "in the game" without the use of all his muscles. The body responds by calling on other muscles to take over the load. (This is called *muscle substitution*.) It's like a football game where the quarterback tries to play center as well as quarterback. The team is incomplete. They may be able to finish the play, but the possibility of injury has increased. The team doesn't function well without one of its players, just as the knee, or any other joint, doesn't function well without its supportive muscles. This causes the other muscles to be used inefficiently, possibly causing a stress-type injury to the joint.

Immediate treatment is the best method for dealing with a contusion: Rest, Ice, Compression and Elevation (commonly known as "*R.I.C.E.*"). This results in less bleeding into the tissue, lessening the severity of the injury. Certainly R.I.C.E. should be followed for the first 48 to 72 hours. Massage should **never** be used at this stage. The goal here is to restrict the motion. Rest the affected area and ice it. This decreases bleeding and swelling by causing the blood vessels to constrict. Use compression on the area, such as wrapping with an Ace bandage. This also restricts further bleeding. Elevation means keeping the limb higher than the heart, decreasing blood pressure in the area, which also helps decrease bleeding.

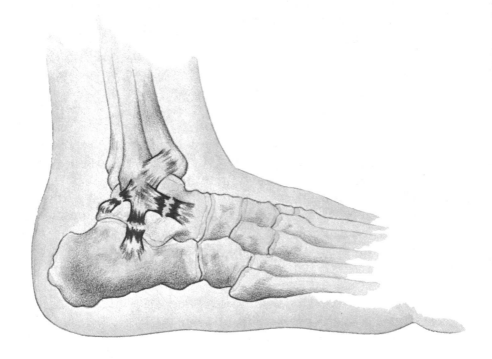

*Ankle Sprain. The ankle ligaments on the lateral aspect of the
ankle in this case are torn.*

## LIGAMENT SPRAINS

A <u>sprain</u> is a tear of a ligament. This can either be a
partial tear or a complete tear. Sprains are graded in degrees
according to severity, first-degree being minimal, second-degree
moderate, and third-degree severe. Tears of the ligament are
usually due to *distraction* (pulling apart) injuries. Forcibly
exceeding the normal range of motion of a joint will tear the
ligament, resulting in a sprain.

Complete dislocations of all joints result in third-degree
sprains of the ligaments and capsules surrounding the joints. It
is important not to get this confused with the word *strain*—the

only difference being that when the word "sprain" is mentioned, it is a ligament injury and when "strain" is mentioned, it refers to a muscle or tendon tear or injury.

## ANATOMY OF THE MUSCLE

Other types of injuries to muscles are called *strains* which can vary in degree of severity. To understand strains, we need to review the anatomy of the muscle. Muscle makes up about 40% of the body weight in men and slightly less than that in women. Muscle is connected to bone by a tendinous structure and has an *origin* and *insertion.*

The nerve enters the muscle and the impulses in the nerve cause the muscle to contract. Without nerve impulses, muscles would not contract.

Skeletal muscles have thousands of narrow muscle cells. These are the contracting elements. The muscle fibers work by shortening and lengthening.

We think of muscle contraction as shortening, but the lengthening type of contraction is just as important. Muscles may also contract as they lengthen. In squatting, when you gradually bend your knee, all the muscles in front of the thigh (*the quadriceps*) are lengthening while the muscles behind the knee (*the hamstrings*) are shortening. If you reverse the process, suddenly standing up, the quadriceps are shortening and hamstrings are lengthening. The muscles that are working the hardest against gravity will be contracted the most, so the quadriceps muscles will be working the hardest, both in squatting and standing up.

There are technical terms for these types of contractions. The lengthening type is called an *eccentric contraction*, while the shortening type is called a *concentric contraction*. Certain types of muscle strengthening exercises will use the eccentric contraction while other types of muscle strengthening exercises will use concentric contractions.

Muscle attaches to tendon as it nears the bone, and the tendon then attaches to the bone. The junction where the muscle forms into the tendon is called the "muscle-tendon junction" (*musculotendinous junction*). The mid-portion of the muscle, the bulky part, is called the *muscle belly.*

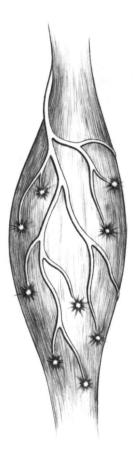

*Nerve Impulse. This is an example of the nerve entering the muscle, providing stimulation to the muscle which causes the muscle to contract.*

The *fascia* is a strong, fibrous tissue which gives support and holds together soft tissues such as muscles, tendons, nerves and blood vessels. It is like a webbing throughout the body, surrounding and holding as well as forming a shock absorption layer. Each muscle is surrounded by these tough, fibrous fascia called *muscle sheaths*.

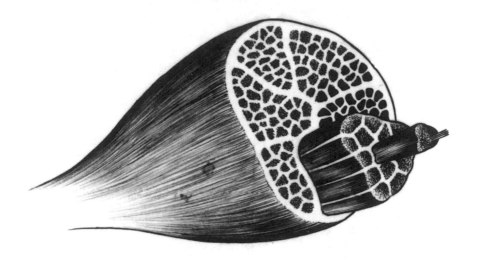

*This is a cross section of the muscle showing the muscle fibers and fibrils.*

## MUSCLE INJURIES

When an injury to the muscle happens, sometimes bleeding will occur within the muscle and the muscle sheath, causing an increase in pressure. Eventually the bleeding will be stopped due to the increase in pressure. If the muscle sheath is damaged, the blood <u>leaks out</u> between the other muscles, causing a *hematoma*. A bleeding that is <u>confined</u> by the muscle sheath or fascia is also a *hematoma*—one that can be very troublesome because the increased pressure within the muscle sheath can cause enough decrease in blood flow that the muscle itself loses its blood flow. This is called a *compartment syndrome*. Compartment syndromes are usually very painful, causing a limited range of motion. Any stretching of that muscle causes severe pain. If a compartment syndrome is suspected, a health professional should be consulted immediately.

## STRAINS

When you understand this basic anatomy, it is easier to understand *muscle strains*, or the tearing of the muscle fibers. It can be a complete muscle rupture or a minor strain, where only a few of the fibers are torn. When the fibers are torn, bleeding occurs. This results in a hematoma. The immediate treatment is the same as for contusions—R.I.C.E.

As many as a third of all sports injuries are attributed to muscle injuries. They tend to heal in about three weeks, especially if R.I.C.E. is applied *immediately*.

When an injury occurs caused by a forceful pull of the muscle, sometimes, instead of the muscle or the tendon attached to it rupturing, the tendon pulls away, taking with it a piece of bone. This is called an *avulsion fracture*.

Ruptures where the muscles are pulled apart from each other are called *distraction ruptures*. These are most common in the explosive types of sports: football, soccer, basketball, jumping and sprinting.

## HAMSTRING PULL

A *hamstring pull* is a muscle tear or rupture of varying degrees. It can be disabling for many weeks. Injuries of this type are more frequently seen in those muscles which cross two joints (as opposed to muscles which cross only one joint). The hamstring muscles are more prone to this type of injury than other muscles because the hamstring muscles cross both the hip joint and the knee joint.

## HEALING A MUSCLE STRAIN OR A RUPTURE

With strains or ruptures, the torn ends of the muscle retract and the area is filled with blood. At this point the body begins an attempt to heal itself. First, it begins to reabsorb some of the blood. Then it follows up with a repairing process by forming fibrous scar tissue. This new muscle tissue regenerates very quickly and easily, but the new muscle fibers will be shorter and incorporate scar tissue that lacks the contractile features of a true muscle tissue, so it will not contract as easily. If it is a severe injury to a muscle, with most of the muscle retracted and with much of the defect filled in with non-contractile scar tissue, the muscle will lose a great deal of its capability for adequate contraction. This leaves it weaker and prone to another rupture.

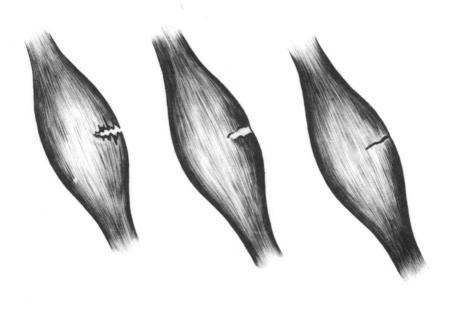

*a. A muscle tear b. Healing muscle tear, filling in with blood and fibrous tissue. c. Healed muscle tear. The tear is filled in with fibrous issue.*

It is important in severe muscle tears to have the muscle repaired surgically by pulling the contracted ends together, so that the area gap and therefore the amount of scar tissue between the muscles is minimized. Complete tears of the musculotendinous junction should almost always be surgically repaired.

## TENDINITIS

*Tendinitis* is the inflammation of the tendon or, frequently, inflammation around the tendon. Often, inflammation of the tendon or the tendon sheath is caused by repetitive micro tears of the tendon due to the overload or overuse of the tendon. Treatment for this kind of condition involves treating the cause of the overload and tearing of the tendon, as well as treating the inflammation itself. In general, areas of inflammation are treated with rest, ice and anti-inflammatory medication such as aspirin. Sometimes injections are used in areas of severe inflammation.

Tendon tears can vary in degrees, in much the same way as muscle tears. There are first-degree, second-degree and third-degree tendon tears. Frequently, a first degree tear can be called tendinitis. A small tear of the tendon can be healed by inflammation and scar tissue the same as a muscle tear. Many small tears, such as the type that happens with the rotator cuff tendinitis—seen in the shoulder—can develop into a complete tear or rupture. Tendon rupture frequently occurs in areas where the blood supply is limited, such as in the mid-portion of the Achilles tendon. Such small tears and inflammation lead to a weakening of the tendon. Then a sudden pull from the strong calf muscle can cause a rupture in an already-weakened Achilles tendon, requiring surgical repair. (*See Chapter Eight, Focus on the Foot.*)

There are predisposing factors which make the tendon more susceptible to injury. One is when tension is applied to the tendon with great force and without adequate warm-ups.

Another factor which contributes to tendon injuries is when the muscle has built up strength faster than the tendon. In other words, the muscle strength is out of proportion to the tendon or tendon attachment strength. This can contribute to both complete tears of the tendon or complete avulsion of the tendon (pulling the tendon off of the bony attachment.) This also contributes to small tears in the tendon, resulting in inflammation and tendinitis. **Since muscle strengthens faster than tendon,** it is common to see this type of injury, where the muscle actually pulls off the tendon attachment. This needs to be repaired surgically.

## PARTIAL TENDON RUPTURE

Partial rupture of the tendon, first- and second-degree tears, can be of an <u>acute</u> (comes on quickly) or a <u>chronic</u> (goes on for a long time) nature. An acute partial rupture begins suddenly, with a specific event, whereas a chronic rupture is often due to a gradual onset of pain. The partial tears occur in the Achilles tendon, the patellar tendon, the rotator cuff and the biceps tendon.

If partial ruptures are not treated appropriately, they can lead to chronic inflammation of the area and further tearing of the tendon. If recognized and treated appropriately, these can heal without further pain and inflammation and without further damage to the tendon. Therefore, it is important to distinguish between a partial rupture and an acute inflammation.

## COMPLETE TENDON RUPTURES

Complete tendon ruptures are common in older athletes who have recently returned to activity without properly training first. This can happen when the person's tendon is degenerative or already in a weakened condition due to chronic inflammation. Therefore, a sudden return to forceful activity can rupture the tendon. Or, the tendon may be healthy but the athlete returns too quickly to activity before it has a chance to build up to normal strength. Although it may not be an abnormal tendon to start off with, it has simply been weakened from lack of use and cannot take the amount of force that is demanded when the athlete returns to a more active lifestyle. Normally, the complete rupture is a noticeable event, in that a painful "snap" is felt, accompanied by a loss of motion in the effected joint.

Normally, this type of injury is surgically repaired, and certainly should be seen by a specialist as soon as possible. This injury is especially common in contact sports and in *ballistic sports*—such as racquetball and handball—sports requiring quick, sudden movements, necessitating quick, forceful contraction of the muscle.

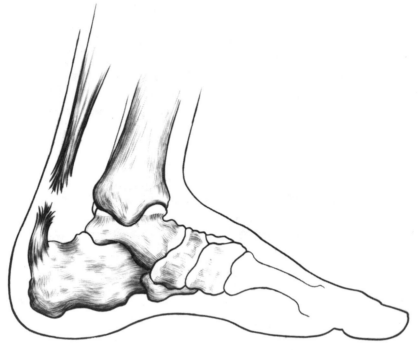

*A complete Achilles rupture. This is usually surgical repaired.*

## INFLAMMATION

The body's response to tissue injury is *inflammation*. The tissue injury can be caused by overload or repeated microscopic injury to the musculoskeletal system. It can also be caused by pressure or friction and external trauma. Inflammation can even be caused by infection.

The inflammatory process is a complex biological response which involves cellular and enzyme changes in the specific area involved. It is the body's attempt to break down and remove the injured tissue, filling it in with scar tissue. If treated appropriately, the inflammatory process can heal the injury. Otherwise, there can be more inflammation, more breakdown and further limitation of function and weakening of the tissue over a period of time. This is called *chronic inflam-*

*mation*. Chronic inflammation takes longer to treat and heal than acute inflammation.

*Acute inflammation* is when there is one injury and the body responds to that injury. When this occurs, there will be increased blood flow to the area, warmth, pain and decrease in function. **This inflammatory response can be decreased if acted upon quickly.** The sooner the acute injury is treated by icing, decreasing the bleeding in the area, and limiting the amount of further injury, the more the inflammatory response will be decreased. **The sooner it is treated, the sooner the injury will heal, and less scar tissue will be formed.**

Inflammation can be caused by friction due to external causes such as poorly fitted shoes, as well as by overuse. This causes a breakdown of the tissue. An example of this is the blisters so many athletes unfortunately develop.

When the suffix *"itis"* is seen at the end of a word, it means *inflammation*. The first part of the word will tell the location of the inflammation. For example, *bursitis* is an inflammation of the bursa; *tendinitis*, inflammation of the tendon; "Arthro" is taken from the Greek reference to "joint" (arthron), so *arthritis* means inflammation of a joint.

## BURSITIS

Frequently, *bursitis* is caused by friction irritation. The bursa are small sacs lined with synovial tissue which secrete fluid as a lubricant. The bursa lie between two areas of the body, allowing smooth movement and sliding of those tissues over each other. They are frequently found between a bone and a tendon, between two tendons and, often, they are located over a bony prominence close to the skin, allowing the skin to move smoothly over the bony prominence. To better understand this, picture a bursa lying between the kneecap and the skin. It can easily be palpated and allows the skin to move smoothly over the kneecap. Pressure or frictional stress on these bursas may lead to inflammation (bursitis).

In this case, it is necessary to treat the bursitis with anti-inflammatory medication to decrease the inflammation and determine and eliminate the cause as well. Bursitis in the athlete can also be caused by infection. This needs to be treated professionally to eliminate both the infection and the cause.

## MUSCLE CRAMPS

Muscle cramps are often encountered in individuals engaged  in vigorous ballistic types of sports (fast stop-and-go movements like aerobics, football and handball). These cramps are often seen in the muscle bellies, more particularly in the calves. Muscle cramps are not caused by *electrolyte imbalance*, but may be due to inadequate *hydration* (not enough fluid intake). Failure to warm-up or stretch properly, or running faster than you have trained to can also lead to cramps.

Cramps generally occur with athletes early in the season, when they have yet to reach proper conditioning. When a cramp occurs, the person should stretch the muscle if possible—a nice, gentle stretch. This should relieve the cramping. If the cramping persists or recurs, consult an athletic trainer or a physical therapist.

## MUSCLE SORENESS

Muscle soreness happens with most new forms of physical activity.  More than likely, it is due to micro tears of the tissue, as in a first-degree muscle strain. Within 24 to 72 hours of new activity, the body is sore and is rebuilding micro-damaged tissue that has been mildly strained. This is a self-limiting condition that leaves in a matter of days as the athlete continues to progress in proper conditioning. During this time, gentle exercise is recommended. If soreness persists beyond the 72-hour time frame, it may be an injury that is significant and needs attention.

## SKELETAL INJURIES OR INJURIES TO THE BONE

Injuries to the bone that result in a break are called *fractures*. Fractures may be oblique, spiral, comminuted or traverse. These fractures are illustrated on the following page, and should be self-descriptive.

Fractures are frequently caused by direct trauma as well as twisting injuries or loss of balance. An *oblique* or *spiral fracture* is caused by a twisting injury. Spiral fractures are common in skiing, especially when the bindings fail to release in a fall. Fortunately, with newer and safer ski equipment, these fractures are happening less and less.

When we hear the word *fracture*, we think it means only a slight crack. This is not so. **A fracture is a break in the bone, and it is serious.** There are degrees of severity in fractures, which can be determined by the use of an x-ray. Fractures in children are different from fractures in adults, because in children the bones are still growing. Because of this, it is important that fractures in children be treated by a specialist to avoid secondary problems such as growth disturbances.

When the fracture pierces the skin, it is called a *compound fracture* or *open fracture*. This almost always requires surgery to repair and prevent bone infection. An *avulsion fracture* is when a ligament pulls a piece of bone loose. This happens most frequently in adolescents, since their muscles and ligaments are stronger at this time than the bone. However, avulsion fractures are found in the adult athlete as well. Occasionally these are repaired surgically.

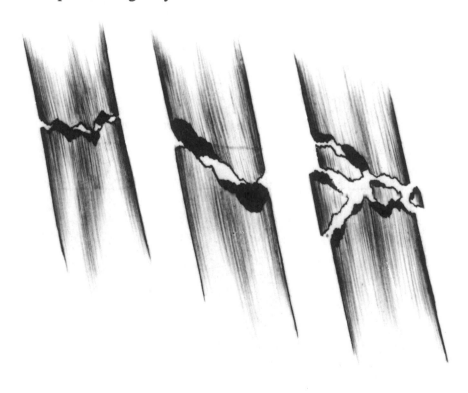

*Complete fractures of bone. a. Transverse fracture*
*b. Oblique fracture c. Comminuted fracture.*

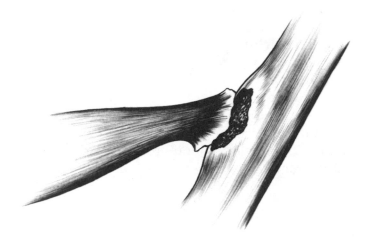

*Avulsion fracture. The tendon is pulled off from the bone, taking with it a piece of the bone. X-ray shows a fractured ankle which has been surgically repaired called open reduction internal fixation.  a. Anterior/posterior view of the ankle.  b. A lateral view of the ankle.*

An important thing to know about fractures is that the soft tissue around the fracture, the muscle, blood vessels, tendons, etc., are also injured when the bone is broken. Broken bones must always be seen by the physician for appropriate evaluation and treatment. The bone may need to be properly set, so that it, as well as the surrounding area, can be allowed to heal properly. We call this reducing the fracture, or *fracture reduction*. The fractured bone also needs to be held in place, or *immobilized*. This can be done by a cast treatment or by surgical fixation of the bone—called *internal fixation*. Sometimes a fracture cannot be put back in place properly without surgery. This simply means that the bone had to be surgically put together using either screws, plates, wires, rods, etc. which are designed especially for the purpose, and are made from specialized stainless steel metals. This is called *open reduction-internal fixation*.

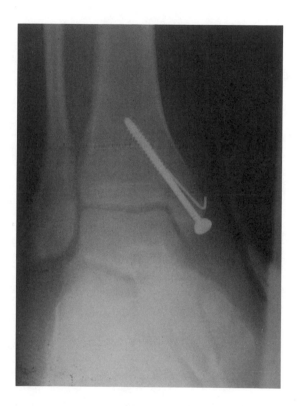

*X-ray of ankle after open reduction-internal fixation for a fractured ankle.*

Whole fields of medicine are devoted to the study and treatment of fractures, and volumes of books have been written on this subject. Fractures are not to be taken lightly, and should be seen by your physician as quickly as possible and treated by a specialist.

## DISLOCATIONS

A *dislocation* means that the two articular surfaces of a joint, previously in contact with each other, have been completely separated and no longer have contact. This means that part of the capsule and part of the ligaments are torn.

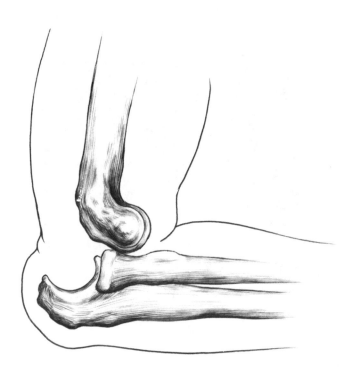

*A complete dislocation of the elbow joint.*

In the case of a complete dislocation, it must be appropriately reduced and the capsule and ligaments which were torn must be treated. This sometimes requires surgery and a rehabilitation program.

In the case of a dislocated shoulder, a brace or a sling may be used for immobilization. A partial dislocation is called a *subluxation*, meaning that the joint only partially went out. In this case, the joint will spontaneously go back into place. This is frequently seen in unstable knees where the kneecap will go out and then come back in. In the case of a knee that has a torn ligament, there is a subluxation called a *rotatory instability*. This recurrent subluxation, if allowed to continue, can cause a wear-and-tear of the articular surface that can eventually lead to *arthritis* of the joint. To prevent this and to stabilize the joint, surgery is sometimes necessary.

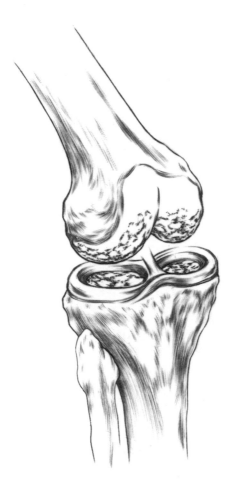

*Arthritic knee showing the breakdown of the cartilage surface due to repeated "wear and tear."*

## STRESS INJURIES

Stress injuries follow certain biomechanical principles. It's a simple rule. Tissue, whether soft tissue—tendons, ligaments, muscles, cartilage, etc., or bone, will break down when a force is imposed on it that exceeds its limit of strength. Strength, of course, varies according to the type of tissue and its density. Whether it breaks or not depends on the type of force applied. Direct trauma (one major force) or many smaller forces that exceed the strength of the tissue can cause it to break.

We can compare the body tissue to a coat hanger. The coat hanger will hold up a coat just as our musculoskeletal system will hold us up. If you try to tow a car with a coat hanger, it will break. If you hit it with an axe, it will be cut in two with one blow. That would be an example of one force causing the breakdown of the material (direct trauma). Similarly, if we're hit by a car, tissues break (direct trauma).

Now apply the same reasoning, using many small loads to break the coat hanger. We know that if we bend the coat hanger repeatedly, it will eventually break. **Repeated small traumas which exceed the strength of the area over a long period of time cause a breakdown of the tissue.** In bone this is called a *stress fracture*. Just like the coat hanger, the bone weakens and eventually breaks.

## STRESS FRACTURES

Stress fractures frequently occur due to repeated overloading of the skeleton over a long period of time. Overloading of the bone causes micro fractures which may develop into complete fractures. *Micro fractures* are slight cracks in the surface of the bone and do not always show up on an x-ray.

Sometimes a *bone scan* is needed to diagnose a stress fracture. The bone breakdown causes a higher rate of turnover of calcium and phosphate in the area of stress fracture. With a bone scan, radioactive phosphorous is injected into the body. A few hours later it will show up as an increase in radioactivity at the area of the stress fracture. This is detected by sophisticated scanning instruments. This is not dangerous. You don't glow in the dark.

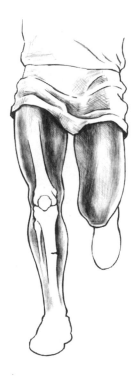

*Illustration of a runner, showing a stress fracture of the tibia.*

Micro fractures may finally result in a *complete stress fracture*. Complete stress fractures are often more severe than complete fractures (caused by direct trauma) in the same area. In direct trauma, the bone is healthy prior to breaking. In a complete stress fracture situation, the micro fractures have caused a chronic condition which has essentially left the bone unhealthy. Stress fractures often occur because too much load or too much stress is absorbed by the bone instead of the muscle system. In other words, the muscles are not taking their share of the load, forcing the skeletal system to take more than its share, and causing an over-stress to the bone and chronic breakdown.

Some of the predisposing factors that contribute to stress fractures are inadequate flexibility and lack of coordination. Because of lack of flexibility, there is not enough movement in the joint to help to absorb shock. If the muscles are not functioning properly, such as in lack of coordination, the body movement is inefficient and the shock is not being properly absorbed, so stress fractures or stress injuries may occur. This can also happen if the muscle involved lacks proper endurance, coordination or flexibility for what it is being asked to do. These are called the *intrinsic factors*.

*Extrinsic factors* which contribute to stress fractures might be improper shoes, poor shoe wear, poor shock absorption, other improper equipment, or improper running or playing surfaces.

A diagnosis of stress fracture should be considered when there is a persistent pain over a weight-bearing bone in any athlete. Although stress fractures are frequently seen in the beginning athlete, they are seen in the well-trained and the professional as well.

## OTHER SPORTS-RELATED INJURIES
### LACERATIONS – CUTS

Lacerations, or cuts, are frequently seen in the athlete during competition. Abrasions and puncture wounds are also often seen. Immediate treatment of open wounds is done by elevating the injured area, applying direct pressure to impede bleeding, and applying a pressure dressing. Cleaning the wound is especially important, and deep wounds should be seen by a doctor or treated at a medical facility as soon as possible (within six hours). **The longer the wound is left open and dirty, the greater the chance of infection.** A wound that has been open for about six hours, or one that is very dirty should not be sutured closed immediately. It is best to treat lacerations as soon as possible.

### BLISTERS

Once a blister has formed, it should not be broken deliberately except with a sterile instrument. When a blister is broken, it is important to apply an antiseptic solution.

Of course, prevention of blisters is more to the point. Many runners and recreational athletes find that using Vaseline$^R$ on their feet can help protect against the rubbing and friction that causes blisters. If you are planning on participating in running as a fitness activity, it's best to break in a pair of new running shoes by walking around in them for a few hours before going out on your first short run. That way your feet will become acclimated to the feel of that particular shoe.

One first-time marathoner made the mistake of wearing brand new shoes, brand new socks and coating his feet with a layer of powder on marathon morning. Before the race was three miles old, he had accumulated, on each foot, a collection of blisters the size of a small mobile home park. As you can imagine, the rest of his marathon was not a very pleasant experience.

The best prevention is to wear good gear, including good quality shoes and socks. If needed, areas of the foot or hand should be padded with an adhesive prior to exercise, to prevent rubbing of sensitive areas of the skin. This is especially true of the hands of athletes who compete in wheelchairs. Other aids that some athletes may need to use, such as artificial limbs, or even playing sports while sitting in chairs or on the floor for long periods of time can cause irritation and even blisters or sores. Daily close inspection is advised so that blisters or sores can be seen and treated immediately.

## RUNNER'S PAIN

Have you ever gone jogging every day with your friends at, say, a 9-minute-per-mile pace, then shown up at a local 10k race and tried to run a lot faster? Can you say, "I-got-a-big-cramp-on-the-side-of-my-belly-and-could-barely-walk boys and girls?" Somehow I knew that you could.

Runners often feel a sharp pain in the upper abdomen either on the right or the left side, just below the diaphragm. One theory is that this is caused by a lack of oxygen supply to the diaphragm. Another is that this is brought on by running too soon after eating and that you should try to avoid running right after meals—wait for a few hours instead. Some feel that this can be brought on if you run at a faster pace than your body is accustomed to. That way, while running daily at a slower pace, the intercostal muscles in the diaphram, between the ribs, are never taxed. Then, all of a sudden, you run faster than your body has been trained to do and you breathe, trying to use those muscles, but they just won't kick in and then *they begin to cramp up.*

It is felt that this can be avoided with breathing exercises which strengthen those muscles as well as gradually increasing running speed during training, and not waiting until the day of the race. Don't ask your body to do what it is not trained to do. If you intend to run fast, gradually train your body to meet that goal.

If runner's pain should occur, remember that this pain does not necessarily mean that you are out of the race. Stop running, bend forward, relax and breathe evenly. It may go away and you can still finish the race.

**But sometimes, believe it or not, it's better not to finish the race.** In the heat of competition, or just plain working out, many people forget that the fitness race doesn't end with that particular run, bike ride or neighborhood basketball game. Hopefully, fitness is something you will savor and enjoy for the rest of your life. That's why it is so important to keep close tabs on your body and to be aware of any pain or nagging injury that, if not nipped in the bud, could put you on the unable-to-work-out-list for an extended period of time. **Listen to your body.** If it's telling you it's time to rest or that it's time to find out what's causing a particular pain, DO IT! Remember that the name of the game is *Lifetime Fitness* and that to score ...you've got to stay in the starting lineup!

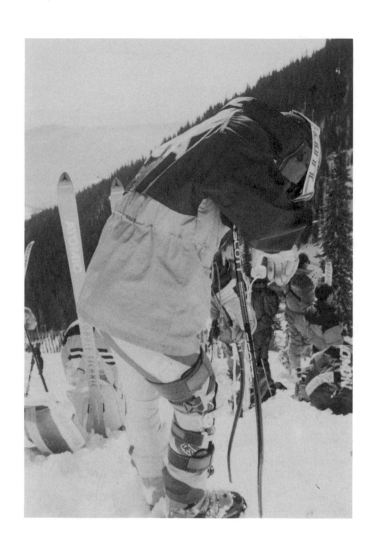

# The Knee

# The Knee

"The knee bone's connected to..."

"Shhh! Quiet, Bunky! I'm trying to concentrate on this knee stuff. And one thing's for sure, if you get a knee injury, you won't be humming a tune. You'll be singing the blues!"

## SPORTS-RELATED KNEE INJURIES

The human knee functions as a combination joint with a hinge-like action that also has the ability to rotate slightly. The *tibia* (the shinbone you can feel at the front and center of your lower leg) and the *femur* (the thighbone) meet to form the knee. The femur's lower end and the tibia's upper end come together in a hinged socket. The top of the shinbone has two rounded hollows, like a cup, while the thighbone has matching protrusions. The two bones fit snugly together and form a tight union with the help of ligaments and cartilage. A form-fitting pad of cartilage, called *meniscus*, surrounds the joint on each side (both medial—inner side, closer to the middle; and lateral—the outer side). The two menisci have several important functions; primarily they add stability to the joint throughout the range of motion and help distribute weight in the joint.

The ligaments on each side of the joint, along with the joint capsule, restrain the joint from rocking from side to side (*valgus* and *varus stress*). These are called the *collateral ligaments* and are outside the joint.

While the medial collateral (MCL) and lateral collateral ligaments keep the knee stable from side to side, the two ligaments inside the knee, called the *cruciate ligaments*, keep the knee from moving excessively from front (anterior) to back (posterior). These two ligaments are called the cruciate ligaments because they cross inside the knee—the *anterior cruciate ligament* (ACL) in front and the *posterior cruciate* in back.

The ligaments are most important in providing the *passive stability* of a joint (stability without muscle control). The bone contour with its cartilage covering and the form-fitting menisci also add to the joint's passive stability.

In addition to the passive stability provided by the ligaments, cartilage and bone, the muscles provide the active stability. The quadriceps muscles that straighten or extend the knee and the hamstring muscles that flex the knee give the knees *active stability*. When the muscles are relaxed there is no active stability. Therefore symptomatic joint looseness or instability results when the ligaments are torn or stretched.

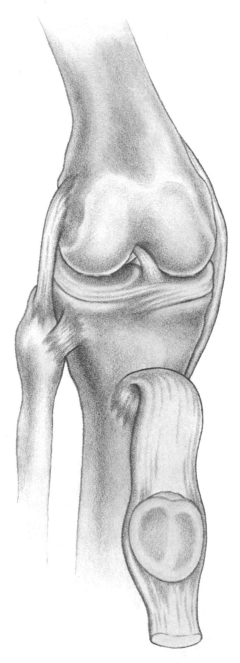

*In this illustration of the knee, the quadriceps tendon and the patella, or kneecap, have been removed in order to see the ligaments and cartilage inside the joint. The muscles and joint capsule have been removed. The thick fibrous bands shown on the outside of the knee are the collateral ligaments.*

The human knee is the single largest weight-bearing joint in the body and is vulnerable to injury. Any sport that involves quick starts, sudden directional changes, jumping, twisting, abrupt stopping or forceful contact is a primary source of knee injury. A sudden blow to the side of the leg can cause injury to the knee, either to the ligaments, meniscus or both. Sports injuries of the ligaments in the knee most frequently affect either the medial collateral or the anterior cruciate ligaments.

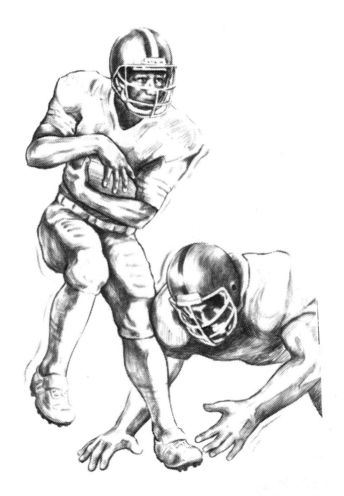

*Football player being clipped, which can result in a knee injury common to contact sports. This is an example of a direct trauma injury, a blind-sided direct hit from another player, causing ligament damage.*

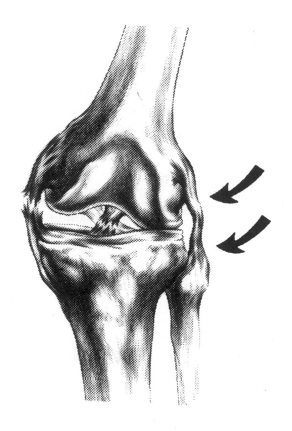

*A torn anterior cruciate ligament and a torn medial collateral ligament. This is a frequent injury seen after a clipping type injury previously illustrated.*

The external ligaments are called *medial collateral* and *medial capsular ligaments* and *lateral collateral* and *lateral capsular ligaments*. They have different sources of blood supply than the ligaments inside the joint. Injury to these ligaments is the typical "knee sprain."

First-degree sprain—minimal

There is usually slight swelling and pain. In some cases, bracing or immobilization is necessary. But, sometimes the athlete is playing a week or so later.

Second-degree sprain

The ligament is significantly torn. Some instability of the joint is present due to the laxity of the injured ligaments. More pain, swelling and limitation of motion is present. The athlete's knee is frequently placed in a brace or immobilized for four to six weeks. If not treated properly, the knee may end up loose, due to the ligament laxity and will require surgery.

Third-degree sprain

A complete tear of the ligament. It may be treated with a brace, but surgery is often required. Neglecting treatment of a third-degree tear will result in severe problems in the knee.

## ACL

The ACL (Anterior Cruciate Ligament) is very important to knee stability and is frequently injured during sports events either as an isolated tear or in combination with other ligaments and the meniscus. For instance, when the knee is injured in skiing, 65% of the time the ACL is torn. Complete tears of the ACL are actually more frequent than partial tears. Complete tears of the ACL do not heal, due to the loss of blood supply to the torn ligament. Even partial tears of the ACL can develop into complete tears due to the lack of blood supply. When the injury occurs, the ligament is stretched, tearing some or all of the fibers—which lose their blood supply and die. This leaves the knee without a functioning ACL.

The ACL is essential to anterior stability of the knee. Attaching from the back part of the femur to the front part of the tibia inside the joint, it is the main guard that keeps the tibia from sliding forward when the knee is bent. When the ligament is torn, instability and looseness results. In technical terms, this is called *rotatory instability*, either medial or lateral.

Rotatory instability is one of the most common problems in sports knee injuries. Without the ACL, the knee often gives out or shifts out of place when the body rotates. A sudden change of direction while running or a cutting-type movement will cause the knee to give way. In other words, if the foot is planted, making the lower leg fixed while the upper body and thigh make a sudden shift or change in direction, the lower leg will fail to follow the shift in direction, and the knee will give out.

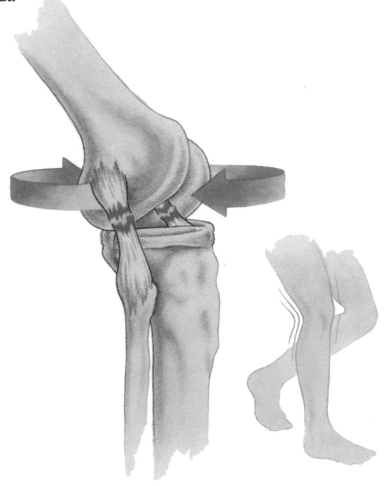

*Rotatory instability of the knee frequently results after an untreated tear of the anterior cruciate ligament. In this illustration, the right foot is planted and the person rotates to the right side. The lower leg does not follow the upper body because of the knee ligament laxity, causing the knee to partially sublux.*

Treatment for this injury depends on the degree of looseness, the amount of instability, and the possibility that other structures might be involved. Treatment is also dependent upon the future demands the athlete wishes to make of his or her body.

Some people, by avoiding activities that cause the knee to give out, can function well without surgery. Some can even have limited sports participation, depending on the degree of laxity of the knee. Strengthening the muscles and bracing are helpful in those who elect not to have surgery.

If the instability is untreated, the continued episodes of subluxation cause injury and eventually the breakdown of the cartilage inside the joint. Over the years this may lead to degenerative arthritis.

With the breakthroughs in arthroscopic surgical techniques as well as rehabilitation, more and more athletes are electing to go the surgical route. With the newer techniques, there is less scarring, less pain, earlier motion to the joint and easier rehabilitation.

The surgery provides either repair or replacement of the ligament. When the indicated surgery is done, there is a high success rate in both stabilizing the joint and returning the athlete to full athletic performance.

## POSTERIOR CRUCIATE LIGAMENT

The posterior cruciate ligament prevents the tibia from shifting backward on the femur. An injury to the posterior cruciate is frequently associated with auto injuries, when the knee strikes the dashboard. When the posterior cruciate is torn in sports, most of the time it is caused by a very severe blow, such as hitting full-force on the playing surface, driving the tibia backwards. A severe blow to the front of the leg, causing the knee to hyper-extend, can tear the posterior cruciate.

Of all the injuries sustained at the knee in any sport, the most serious is dislocation. When the knee sustains a blow so powerful that it dislocates, ligaments are torn, and there is sometimes vascular injury which of course restricts vital blood supply.

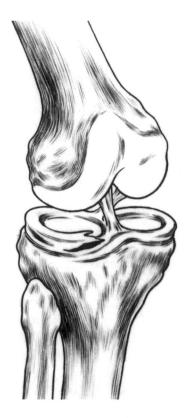

*A tear of the lateral meniscus which interferes with proper joint function. This injury requires arthroscopic surgery.*

## MENISCUS INJURY

Tears of the medial or lateral meniscus (cartilage pads inside the joint) often occur by a weight-bearing, twisting injury. This can either be a direct blow or coordination failure. Sometimes partial tears are seen, which develop into complete tears with repeated episodes of injury. This is true of knees with untreated tears of the ACL that have rotatory instability. When the knee goes out (*subluxation*), pinching the meniscus between the two joint surfaces, this eventually causes a complete tear of the meniscus. It is also common to have more than one tear. Also injuries to the meniscus are often seen as a result of a single injury, as an isolated tear or associated ligament tears.

The clipping injury seen on the earlier page commonly causes the "Unhappy Triad" which is a tear of the ACL, MCL and medial meniscus. In the past, tears of the meniscus were treated with extensive surgery, excising the entire meniscus and repairing the ligaments, followed by a long period of casting and rehabilitation. With the recent development of arthroscopic surgery, all this has dramatically changed. The meniscus function can be preserved either by repair or partial excision. Torn ligaments can be treated more precisely and effectively, shortening rehabilitation time and improving results.

When fragments of torn cartilage are removed arthroscopically, the rim of the meniscus is usually saved and the stability and other functions of the meniscus are preserved. By saving the rim of the meniscus, there is less wear and tear on the joint in the future.

A person with a torn meniscus may experience "locking," in which the knee can't be extended completely; "catching," which feels like there is something caught in the knee; or "giving way," when the knee suddenly collapses or slips. These symptoms are usually caused by the mechanical wedging of the torn piece of cartilage between the two joint surfaces. Repeated episodes of this may cause further damage, effusions (fluid on the knee), and may eventually cause cartilage breakdown.

## ARTHROSCOPIC SURGERY

*Arthroscopic surgery*, a relatively new surgical procedure, is now widely used by orthopedic surgeons. The instrument of focus is an arthroscope, which enables the surgeon to examine the interior of the knee without making large incisions. The technique is used both in diagnosis and treatment of the knee, shoulder, ankle, elbow and wrist. The instrument used consists of a tube about ten inches in length and about as thick as a pencil. It contains optic fibers in the tube which transmit light and become the source of illumination inside the joint and acts as a lens for a small hand-held camera.

In arthroscopic surgery of the knee, with the patient under local or general anesthesia, the arthroscope is inserted into the knee joint through a small incision. Fluid is pumped into the joint to distend it and open up the space for view on a TV screen. The powerful light illuminates the area that comes to view as an image on the screen. The surgeon can move the tip of the arthroscope around in the joint, viewing the entire interior of the joint. By entering the knee with a small probe through another small incision, the surgeon can examine the knee extensively.

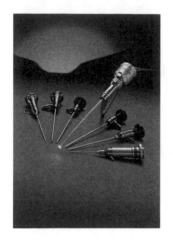
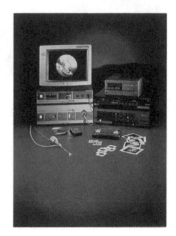

*Arthroscopic Instruments*

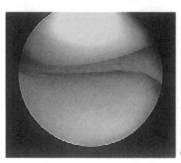
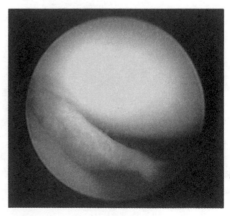

a.                                        b.

*Arthroscopic picture showing: a. Normal cartilage and meniscus*
*b. A torn piece of cartilage wedged between the joint surfaces.*

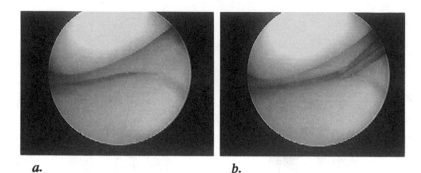

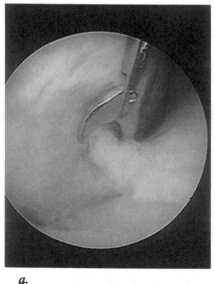
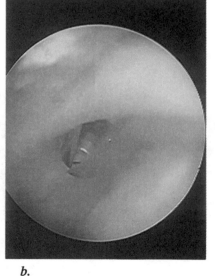

*Arthroscopic picture taken inside the knee joint showing a. Normal meniscus and joint surface. b. Probing the joint with an instrument.*

*Arthroscopic picture showing a. Small scissors cutting scar tissue inside the knee joint. b. Power-cutting rotation suction instrument removing excess scar tissue and loose pieces. Actual size of the instrument is 4.5 millimeters.*

If damage to the inside of the knee is found, the probe is removed and a small surgical instrument is placed into the joint through the same incision. Observing the instrument's position through the arthroscope, the surgeon can perform surgery.

One tool used inside the joint is a small knife used to cut away small bits of tissue that may be growths or fragments. A small scissors is also used to cut small growths that may impair knee function. Tiny chips of cartilage or bone, that may lodge between the joint surfaces and cause pain, can be vacuumed out using a small suction instrument. When the joint has been examined and the needed repairs made, the excess fluid is removed, the scope is withdrawn and the incision taped closed.

Usually the patient has only a very short outpatient hospital stay, compared to the lengthy hospital stay that would be required to recuperate from more extensive surgery. Also, the recuperation time is far less with arthroscopic surgery. The patient can usually walk out of the hospital and physical therapy is often started that day or the day after.

Of course, when there is extensive damage to the knee involving disruption of internal structure, an alternative to arthroscopic surgery may be required. In this case, the knee may be immobilized in a cast or a brace for some weeks after the surgery.

Not all knee injuries require arthroscopic or other forms of surgical treatment. Most overuse injuries can be treated with rest, cessation of athletic activity, ice and/or anti-inflammatory drugs.

### PROBLEMS SURROUNDING THE KNEECAP— THE EXTENSOR MECHANISM: PATELLA, QUADRICEPS, PATELLAR TENDON

The *extensor mechanism* of the knee is composed of the *quadriceps muscles*, the *patella* (the kneecap) and the *patellar tendon*. These three structures—muscle, tendon, and bone—act as a unit. Together they extend or straighten the knee.

The undersurface of the patella is part of the inside of the knee joint. The surface is coated with a layer of cartilage. Whenever the knee moves, the kneecap glides in a groove on the distal end of the femur, also covered with a layer of cartilage. In order for the cartilage surface, which is living tissue, to remain healthy, the patella needs to glide perfectly in the groove with equal pressure on both sides. Unequal pressure will cause deterioration of the cartilage under the kneecap and on the femur, softening of the cartilage and *chondromalacia*, or chronic deterioration of the cartilage of the patella.

In chondromalacia, the cartilage lining the articular surface of the patella softens and forms blisters and cracks and there is fragmentation of the cartilage surface. This ultimately leads to complete breakdown of the cartilage, and arthritis of the patellofemoral joint.

A tire on a car which is out of alignment causes uneven wear. If the patella is not tracking properly, uneven wear on the joint is the result. This uneven tracking of the patella, however, is not the only cause for chondromalacia. Any injury to the articular surface can result in damage to the cartilage. One such injury is direct trauma to the patella, causing injury to the cartilage surface underneath the bone. Another such injury is dislocation of the patella, in which a piece of articular cartilage is damaged as the patella goes completely out of joint. Subluxation of the patella is also a coordination and tracking problem in which the patella partially goes out of joint and causes micro trauma.

Dislocation of the patella is often caused by a coordination failure—the quadriceps muscles on the lateral side of the thigh pull forcefully, pulling the patella out of its groove and dislocating it laterally, tearing the supporting tissue on the medial side. This is more common in females partially because of their increased *Q-angle* (the angle at the knee formed by the extensor mechanism and the lower leg). The wider pelvis found in females contributes to the increased Q-angle. Other predisposing factors such as a shallow groove or a high-riding patella increase the risks of this happening. Dislocation can also be caused by a direct blow to the patella.

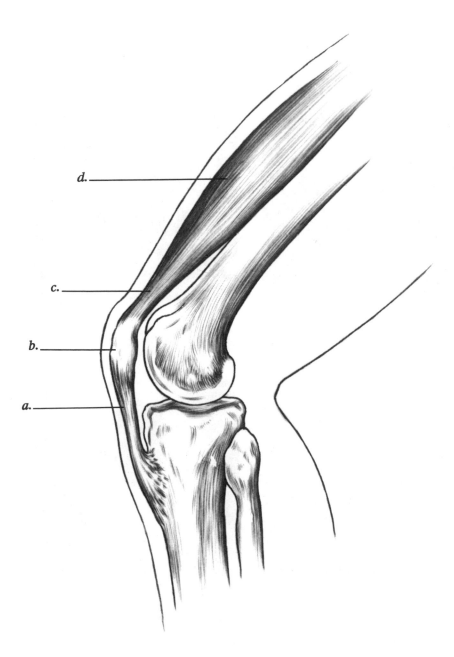

*Lateral view of the knee showing the extensor mechanism a. Patellar tendon b. Patella c. Quadriceps tendon d. Quadriceps muscle. Contraction of the quadriceps muscle extends or straightens the knee joint.*

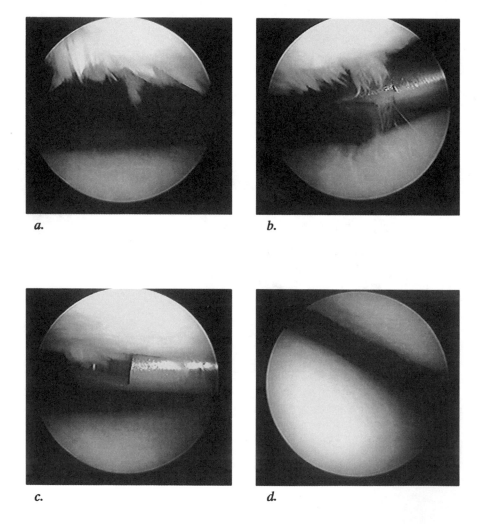

*Arthroscopic picture showing chondromalacia of the patella.*
*a. Notice the rough "crabmeat" above and smooth cartilage*
*surface below. b. Instrument removing the loose cartilage.*
*c. Most of the rough surface has been removed. d. The rough*
*area has been removed.*

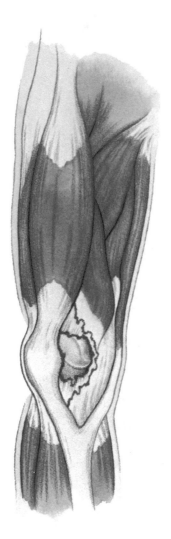

*The quadriceps muscles and patella (extensor mechanism) are shown with the patella dislocated laterally, tearing all the restraining structures on the medial side.*

Any of these factors can cause chondromalacia of the patella, which is a source of pain in the joint felt behind the kneecap with exertion or load on the patella. Frequently, the person with chondromalacia feels pain going down stairs, when squatting, or when sitting for long periods of time. Cracking or grinding of the patella may be felt, but a noisy patella does not necessarily mean chondromalacia. Many times a noisy patella is not painful and therefore does not need treatment.

It is important to remember that pain around the knee-cap, called *patellofemoral pain,* is not always caused by chondromalacia, but chondromalacia can cause pain in the knee.

## OTHER CAUSES OF PAIN AROUND THE KNEECAP

Other conditions which can cause pain around the kneecap are inflammation of the quadriceps tendon, inflammation of the patellar tendon and inflammation of the synovial plica (*plica syndrome*). The inside of the knee joint is lined with the synovium, which secretes synovial fluid. A fold in the synovium, called *synovial plica*, is a normal part of the anatomy of the knee. These folds can become inflamed, causing pain around the kneecap. When this condition becomes chronic, the folds become thickened fibrous bands. Not only can this cause pain, but it can cause catching, locking and giving way of the knee, mimicking a torn cartilage (meniscus). Sometimes surgery is necessary.

Inflammation of the quadriceps tendon just above the kneecap is another cause of pain that needs to be treated with conservative measures. Inflammation of the patellar tendon is sometimes called "Jumper's Knee." This is caused by micro tears in the patellar tendon and sometimes needs to be treated by physical therapy or even by casting.

Inflammation of the attachment of the patella onto the tibia is frequently a cause of pain in the knee. In growing adolescents, it is called Osgood-Schlatter's disease, discussed in *Exercise and the Young Athlete.*

Before treatment, specific identification of the cause of patellofemoral problems should be determined, whether it be chondromalacia, plica syndrome, tendinitis, or other painful conditions. One factor which contributes to most of the patellofemoral problems is a weak muscle (the *vastus medialis obliquus*) called the VMO. This muscle is very important in the last few degrees of extension of the knee and sometimes it gets lazy. A lazy VMO tends to track the kneecap more to the outside and this can cause either chondromalacia or inflammation around the patella, plica syndrome or tendinitis. It is very important to strengthen this muscle and keep it strong through physical therapy exercises.

Another contributing factor to patellofemoral problems is hamstring tightness, which can easily be avoided by proper stretching.

Excessive pronation in the feet can cause more rotation in the tibia, contributing to patellofemoral pain. Anti-inflammatory medications, as well as orthotics, are used in the treatment of this disorder and will be discussed further in the next chapter.

## THIGH INJURIES

Both hamstring and quadriceps injuries are serious since these muscles flex and extend the knee. If there is weakness or lack of flexibility in either, due to an injury or lack of coordination, the knee is left vulnerable to injury. Injured quadriceps can also cause the kneecap not to track properly in it's groove resulting in significant knee pain.

Severe contusion to the quadriceps with bleeding into the muscle and hematoma formation can lead to calcification of the muscle resulting in a permanent loss of part of the muscle function. Thus, muscle and range of motion of the knee can be lost.

It is very important to treat thigh contusions and strains properly, with rest and ice. It is important not to injure the muscle again and cause more bleeding since this is more likely to cause calcification and scar tissue formation. Because of these possible complications, medical attention is necessary for thigh bruises.

## BURSITIS AROUND THE KNEE JOINT

There is a bursa called the *pre-patellar bursa* lying just over the top of the kneecap. It allows the skin to slide over the kneecap. This can become inflamed due to repeated pressure. People who spend a lot of time on their knees, such as carpet layers, can develop markedly swollen, distended, painful and red kneecaps. This can also be caused by an infectious process. Most of the time it is treated conservatively, but occasionally the bursa needs to be excised surgically.

There are other causes of pain around the knee, such as inflammation of the tendon attachments (tendinitis). The most important goal here is to identify the cause as well as the symptoms. The symptoms can usually be treated with anti-inflammatory medication and rest. The cause can be determined by professional examination and treated with coordination, strength and flexibility training.

## FRACTURES IN THE KNEE JOINT

Fractures which actually involve the articular surface of the knee joint are very serious and should always be treated by putting the articular surfaces back together perfectly, usually with surgery. This prevents wear and tear on the cartilage and arthritis later on. An orthopedic surgeon should always evaluate these injuries.

In top shape? Just starting out? World Class Champion or perhaps an Everyday Athlete? No matter, knee injuries do not discriminate. Given the right circumstances, they can strike anyone, anytime, anywhere. The goal, as always, is to stay fit. And to stay fit? You've got to continuously read your body and be aware of any pain or swelling. Remember, sports fans, you can't stay fit if you're out of the game. Protect those knees...they're the only ones you've got!

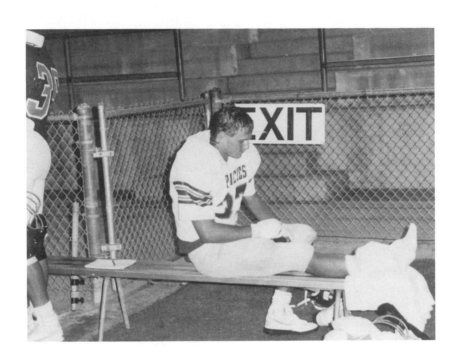

# Focus on the Foot

# Focus on the Foot

Okay, Sports Medicine Fans...It's Quiz Time:
What is the best example of shock?

A) You are audited by the IRS because your tax account-
   ant, who has just left town, claimed in your latest
   return that you have six dependents..., all over 65.
B) You decide to rewire the light socket and, just when
   you are putting all the wires back, someone turns the
   breaker switch on.
C) You run a neighborhood 10k in a pair of cowboy boots
   and later, your feet are sore, your back hurts and you
   notice post-race pain all up and down your lower leg.
D) All of the above.

While the IRS and the light socket can definitely cause
an increase in your adrenaline flow, when we talk real shock,
the foot is where we have to begin.

## How the Foot Works:

The movement of the foot is, as Spock would say, "Fascinating." Whether it is in a contact phase of motion (on the ground), or in a non-contact phase of motion, it needs to be in complete coordination with its counterpart, the other foot, in order to successfully complete forward, backward or any kind of movement without sustaining injury. While in contact with the ground, whether walking, jogging, striding or distance running, the foot goes through three phases. And, no matter which activity is being accomplished (walking, running, etc.), the motion involved in these three phases of the gait cycle remains the same.

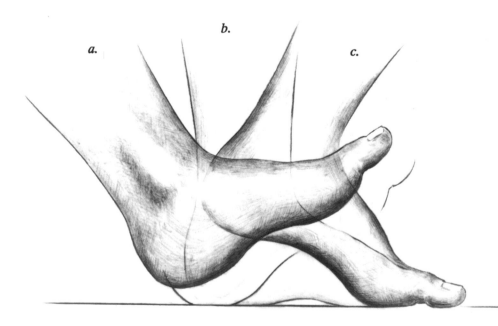

*Phases of the gait cycle. a. Heel strike b. Mid-stance c. Propulsion or push-off.*

The first phase is *heel strike,* when the heel first touches the ground. The second phase is *mid-stance,* when the foot is flat on the ground. The third stage is *propulsion* or push-off, when the foot is pushing off the ground. When the foot leaves the ground, the non-contact phase begins, called the *swing phase* (when the foot is swinging through the air). The foot then goes through another contact cycle when it hits the ground again.

It is important to remember that there are two feet, so when one foot is going through one part of the cycle, the other foot is going through a different part of the cycle. And of course, one foot is always in contact with the ground. Otherwise it would not be called walking or running, it would be considered jumping or leaping through the air.

There have always been many questions from athletes concerning the mechanics of walking and running, as well as the terms *supination* and *pronation,* heard so often in the running community. With a better understanding of these terms and of the foot—a complex part of the body, the athlete can better understand possible foot injuries and may even prevent them from occurring.

## HEEL CONTACT

*Pronation* is normal and natural movement of the foot where the top of the foot rolls inward. This motion helps to loosen the foot up so it can adapt to different ground surfaces. It also enables the joints in the foot to absorb the shock at heel impact. However, excessive pronation, or too much of a roll inward by the top of the foot, leads to more foot mobility than is desirable. Although this still accomplishes shock absorption, excessive pronation leaves the foot unstable. Other muscles, tendons, ligaments and joints try to compensate for this instability and injuries occur. Tendinitis, knee sprain and arch fatigue all result from excessive pronation.

*Pronation* means that the sole of the foot is turned outward and the inside or *medial* part of the foot has contact with the surface. This is a flat foot position. *Supination* means that the sole of the foot is turned inwards, the medial side of the foot is higher than the outside of the foot or that the heel has rolled outward.

At heel contact or heel strike, the foot is usually supinated. Due to the relationship of the hip and leg, the foot will usually strike the ground on the outside portion of the heel. This creates a very unstable platform for the foot, where it can roll inward (pronate) or roll outward (supinate). If the foot rolls outward, it becomes unstable, usually resulting in an ankle sprain.

Seventy-five percent of the time the foot will pronate to where the heel is perpendicular to the ground. The other twenty-five percent, however, tend to *under-pronate*. This means that the foot does not go through enough pronation for normal motion. People with under-pronation tend to have a relatively high arch with a very rigid foot type. This is exactly opposite of a flat foot or over-pronated foot. Because this type of foot is very rigid, it does not absorb shock well. Stability is not a factor, but shock absorption is. Injuries such as heel bruises, stress fractures and shin splints can result from under-pronation and too much shock.

## MID-STANCE

*Mid-stance* is the second phase of the gait cycle, when the foot is in flat contact with the ground. At this point, the foot is ready to accept the body weight, and most of the pronation or supination has already occurred. Since pronation is the normal motion, the foot must resupinate to become more stable and rigid for the next phase. However, too much pronation causes the foot to be too mobile and does not allow it to resupinate. If this should happen, the foot is not in a stable position, which could cause problems.

## PROPULSION OR PUSH-OFF

The last phase of gait is called *propulsion* or push-off. By now the body is using the foot to propel itself forward, and the foot should be in a rigid position through the mechanism of resupination. Without the resupination, the foot cannot be rigid, and the individual must try to push off with a loose and mobile foot. This creates inefficiency as well as shock and jarring in both the *metatarsal* area (long bone area in front of the foot) and in the mid-foot.

Runners often come into my office—their favorite pair of running shoes in hand—concerned because the outside of their running shoes are worn. These athletes think they supinate and may be creating a problem which will result in an injury. Usually, the shoe is worn at the point of normal heel impact. This may not be anything to be alarmed about.

Under-pronation or supination can be seen by a breakdown of the outside of the heel counter and excessive wear on the entire outside aspect of the outer sole of the shoe. Remember that pronation is the *flattening out* of the foot, while supination is the *holding up* of the arch of the foot. Therefore, a very flat foot is a pronated foot, while a foot with a very high arch is a supinated foot.

Excessive pronation can be seen by close observation. A breakdown of the heel counter to the medial side (inside) indicates excessive pronation. Also, sole wear under the ball of the foot indicates excessive pronation or excessive flattening out of the foot.

Both supination and pronation are the normal motions that a normal foot goes through. **It is the extremes of these motions that cause problems.**

## FAR-REACHING EFFECTS OF FOOT PROBLEMS

It is especially important for the health professional to understand these foot mechanics, because **problems in the foot can lead to problems in other parts of the body.** Not enough or too much supination or pronation causes the knee or the hip or even the back to have to compensate. A pain in the knee can be due to over-pronation in the foot. In this case, the knee has to rotate more to compensate, causing a tendinitis or a stress type of injury. Fractures in the foot and lower leg are often caused by poor shock absorption in the foot.

The mechanics of body function is called *biomechanics*. Looking at the biomechanics of a foot, we can compare it to a car tire. The foot absorbs shock just as an inflated tire absorbs shock. If you keep driving on a bumpy road with a flat tire, you're going to cause more problems than just demolishing the wheels. The same is true with the foot. Lack of shock absorption in the foot can certainly cause problems well above the foot. It is not unusual to see athletes who have quit running because of knee pain. They are usually worried that they may never run again or may need knee surgery. Many times all they require is physical therapy and a change of foot mechanics (possibly orthotics). They can then return to running, happy and pain free.

## ANATOMY OF THE FOOT

The foot consists of 26 bones, which are connected by tough ligaments and joint capsules composing about 30 joints. There are also approximately 30 muscles and tendons.

The foot is divided into 3 sections: the heel, the mid-foot and the forefoot. The back part of the foot, or heel, is composed of two bones: the ankle bone, called the *talus*, and the heel bone, or *calcaneus*. These two bones form the hind foot or the back part of the foot. The mid-foot is composed of the middle-sized bones. The front part of the foot, or forefoot, is composed of the *metatarsals*, and the toe bones, or the *phalanges*.

All these bones, plus muscles and tendons, work together:
1. to absorb shock,
2. to propel the foot,
3. to help hold balance during gait.

Many of the tendons which attach into the foot are large muscles in the leg. The lower leg muscles have long tendons which pass in front of and behind the ankle to insert into the bones in the foot. These extend the toes, flex the toes, turn the foot in, turn the foot out, lift the foot up and push the foot. Shorter muscles found in the foot also help control foot motion.

There are two arches in the foot. The long arch is called the *longitudinal arch*, commonly identified as "the arch" of the foot. This extends from the calcaneus to the big toe, or from heel to toe. The other arch is the *transverse arch* which goes across the foot and extends from the ball of the foot on the inside to the little toe ball of the foot. This is called the *transverse arch* or the *metatarsal arch*. The longitudinal arch is supported by the *plantar fascia*.

# PROBLEMS WHICH CAUSE PAIN AROUND THE HEEL

## HEEL BRUISE

Other than the ligaments, tendons and muscles, the most important soft tissue in the foot is the *heel cushion*. This is fat tissue connected with strong fascial connective tissue attached to the skin. This heel pad can break down, getting small tears in the fascia due to excessive pressure on the heel such as a direct blow, causing a sudden rupture of the tissues or a stress-type injury. In this case, the heel has been overused, causing a slow breakdown resulting in a painfully sore heel cushion. Sometimes called a *stone bruise*, this can be treated by taking away excessive pressure, resting the heel, improving the shoe wear to add more shock absorption, and/or adding a heel cup cushion to the shoe.

## STRESS INJURIES

Stress injuries to the foot, just like any other stress or overuse injury, occur when the foot has experienced repeated stress in which microscopic tears and soft tissue injuries occur. The body's inflammatory reaction begins to repair the damaged area. Inflammatory reaction causes pain in the area and, if not treated, can cause a minor injury to develop into a chronically painful area. Stress injuries and even stress fractures frequently occur in the foot. Any persistent pain in this area should be followed by an examination by a medical professional.

## PLANTAR FASIITIS OR HEEL SPUR SYNDROME

*Plantar Fascia* is a thick, fibrous band of tissue which extends from the front part of the heel bone, or calcaneus, forward, fanning out under the arch to the ball of the foot or the *metatarsal head*. Traditionally, the plantar fascia becomes injured through a sudden force exerted on the arch or a chronic, repetitive, excessive pronation or pressure on the arch. Classically, the pain will be felt where the plantar fascia inserts into the calcaneus. Initially, patients will complain of a "stone bruise" or bone bruise immediately below the heel. This can also be confused with an actual bruise to the heel pad or heel cushion.

Irritation of the plantar fascia will generally be more painful the first thing in the morning, and then will warm up within a few minutes. Also, the pain will generally be worse at the beginning of an activity and then feel better during the course of the activity, only to return after a few hours of rest. Examination of the heel by pressing on it with the fingertips can produce a tender area just at the point of insertion of the plantar fascia into the calcaneus.

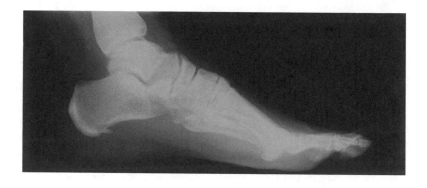

*This lateral x-ray of the foot shows the presence of a bone spur on the heel, or calcaneus bone.*

Sometimes, if the stress across the plantar fascia has existed for a long period of time, a bone spur will develop. If an x-ray is taken it may demonstrate an anterior-looking bone spur beneath the calcaneus pointing in the direction of the plantar fascia. Usually the spur itself doesn't cause the pain. The stress of the plantar fascia on the bone causes pain and inflammation. The spur forms secondarily.

Ice, anti-inflammatory medication and rest are used to treat bone spur inflammation. After relieving the inflammation itself, the cause of the inflammation should be treated. That may require specific exercises to strengthen the foot and to improve coordination, using physical therapy techniques.

Treating the cause may also require support of the foot itself, taking pressure off the longitudinal arch and plantar fascia. Sometimes this can be accomplished with over-the-counter arch supports. Taping may also be used. If the patient responds to taping, but not to the over-the-counter insoles, a custom orthotic device should be made by a professional.

Contributing factors to plantar fasciitis are: tight calf muscles, lack of strength of the muscles in the leg which help to support the arch or the formation of a chronic scar tissue in the area which has not been relieved by a physical therapy modality such as friction massage, ultra sound or immobilization. If all else fails, surgical release of the area is effective.

## "PUMP BUMP" AND BURSITIS

An *exostosis* is a bony growth or bony bump. The bony bumps on the heel are called *"pump bumps."* These are usually found behind the calcaneus and can be extremely painful when pressure is placed over the bumps with shoe gear. Many times a *bursa* will form over the bump, becoming inflamed and causing pain.

Treatment for pump bumps is generally conservative (non-surgical), removing the pressure from the exostosis either through padding the area or padding around the area so there is no direct pressure across the bump. Sometimes a tight Achilles tendon can cause pressure on the bump. In these cases, working on flexibility of the Achilles tendon or calf muscle can help relieve the stress. In extreme cases, surgery is necessary to actually remove the bump.

## POSTERIOR TIBIA TENDINITIS

The *tibialis posterior* muscle is a large muscle in the back of the calf which attaches to a long, thick tendon that extends down behind the *medial malleolus* (inside ankle bone) to the medial arch of the foot. This is a very important muscle/tendon complex. Not only does this muscle help with turning the foot in or inverting the foot, it is also the prime muscle in preventing excessive pronation. It helps support the arch and helps with shock absorption, making it very important in any athletic maneuver in which running is involved.

This tendon frequently becomes inflamed when over-pronation is a problem. Inflammation of the tendon can cause pain in the medial aspect of the ankle and mid-foot, or in the medial aspect of the heel.

Inflammation of the muscle part of this muscle/tendon complex is a common cause of "*shin splints*," which is frequently relieved by reducing the pronation either through arch supports or custom-made orthotics. This treatment is combined with physical therapy to reduce the inflammation and work on strengthening and coordination of the posterior tibial muscle.

## TIBIAL NERVE IRRITATION
## TARSAL TUNNEL SYNDROME

The *tibial nerve* lies very close to the posterior tibial tendon as it moves behind the medial aspect of the ankle. The area in which the tendons, nerves and arteries pass behind the medial aspect of the ankle is covered with a thick fascia to hold the tendons in place. This area is called a *tarsal tunnel*. With excessive foot motion or pronation, this area (where the tendons, nerves and vessels lie) can become irritated, causing inflammation and swelling, tightness where the nerve passes through, and constriction of the nerve. This can result in scarring around the tibial nerve.

The symptom of irritation of the nerve is pain. This pain may mimic that of Achilles tendinitis or posterior tibial tendinitis —and some posterior tibialis or Achilles tendinitis may indeed be present as well. The treatment initially would be conservative: treat the inflammation and the excessive pronation. If symptoms do not resolve with conservative treatment, a closer look into the condition may be necessary to find out if there is severe restriction of the nerve function.

Sophisticated studies directly on the nerve can show its conductivity and whether or not there is any restriction. Severe impairment of the conductivity of the nerve may be an indication for surgery.

# CONDITIONS WHICH CAUSE PAIN IN THE FRONT PART OF THE FOOT OR THE FOREFOOT

## METATARSALGIA

*Metatarsalgia* is one of those wastebasket terms which means pain in the metatarsal region. This is most frequently due to a fallen transverse arch, but it can also occur when one of the metatarsals is in a slightly fallen (or plantar flexed) position.

The transverse metatarsal arch normally allows the majority of the pressure under the forefoot to be transmitted to the fifth and fourth metatarsal heads or from the outside ball of the foot to the inside ball of the foot. Occasionally, however, one of the metatarsal heads becomes plantar flexed or depressed rather than forming a smooth arch. In this case, there is an abnormal distribution of force directly beneath that particular metatarsal head. Pain and sometimes a calloused formation will develop immediately beneath the metatarsal. A weight-bearing x-ray can show the depressed position of that metatarsal. When the foot is palpated, the patient will almost always have the most pain under one particular metatarsal.

Utilization of an *electrodynogram* (a study to analyze stress distribution and gait) with four centers beneath the metatarsal heads will show the one with a significantly higher amount of force.

Frequently the solution to the problem is in the form of padding around the head or using what is called a *metatarsal pad* placed just behind the metatarsal to take pressure off the heads of the metatarsals themselves.

## SESAMOIDITIS

The *sesamoid* bones are two small bones which lie just under the ball of the foot on the great toe side. These are actually small bones which are attached to the tendon which flexes the great toe. They provide leverage for the flexion of the great toe, which is extremely important in gait.

Unfortunately, injuries to these bones are very common. They frequently occur in sports which involve jumping as well as dancing, aerobic dancing and aerobic exercise. Pain around the sesamoid bones is normally diminished with an accommodative pad, sometimes called a "dancer's pad." This accommodation relieves the stress under the first metatarsal phalangeal joint and the sesamoid bones. In difficult or recalcitrant cases, orthotic devices with metatarsal support may be necessary to help lessen the amount of force beneath the first metatarsal.

When fractures of the sesamoids occur, they may apparently heal with no pain in the area. On x-ray they will always show as a fracture, however, since these never heal with formation of new bone, but with a fibrous union instead.

## "MORTON'S NEUROMA"

A *Morton's neuroma* is a build-up of scar tissue around the nerve which passes between two of the metatarsal heads. The nerve generally becomes inflamed either from microtrauma or from a direct trauma insult. In approximately 90% of cases, the neuroma occurs in the third inner space where the two nerves which go to the toes split, going out to the inside of each toe. There will be burning, numbing or radiating pain originating from the third inner space, which travels to the ends of the third and fourth toe. Sometimes the patient will have difficulty identifying the exact digits involved, but usually will experience extreme pain to pressure in the third inner space. The pain will normally be worse in shoe gear, and many times the patient's response to the pain will be to take off their shoes and massage the area. Treatment of this condition is usually to first try pads which fit behind the metatarsal heads, spreading them and decreasing the pressure on the nerve.

If conservative means such as pads, orthotics, injection, and/or a change of shoe wear have not improved the condition, a surgical excision of the neuroma may be necessary.

## PROBLEMS INVOLVING THE TOE

*Turf Toe* is inflammation of the joint of the great toe, an injury to the joint caused by too much sudden flexion of the toe. Pain in this area can also be caused by inflammation around the sesamoid bones or by more severe problems such as gout or other kinds of arthritis. The usual treatment is anti-inflammatory medication and padding the area to reduce the inflammation. Sometimes absolute rest is necessary—yes, even crutches. Not treating the area can lead to a chronic condition which can be disabling.

Severe injury to the first metatarsal joint, such as in repeated injuries in a "turf toe," can result in *Hallux Rigidus*, which means a stiff big toe. This makes it difficult to run because the toe lacks full motion. In cases of turf toe syndrome, the injured athlete should allow at least three to four weeks rest before returning to athletic activity.

## BUNIONS ON THE FOOT

*Bunions* are bony prominences which occur on top or on the sides of the foot. A bunion can increase in size due to both bony build-up and build-up of bursa and scar tissue over the bone. Tight shoe wear often aggravates this condition. The x-rays usually will show the bony prominence or even an extra bone. Like "pump bumps," these areas sometimes have to be removed surgically.

## HALLUX VALGUS

When people talk of bunions, they are often referring to a *Hallux Valgus*. The actual cause of the bunion formation over the inside of the great toe is the condition called Hallux Valgus. This means that the great toe is turning to the outside, creating a greater angle on the inside of the foot at the level of the big toe joint. In this condition, you will usually have a very wide forefoot with the big toe angling outward. The area over the medial aspect of the first metatarsal head becomes prominent and painful in shoe wear. This, then, is called a *bunion*. Treatment can include wearing wider-fitting shoes, padding between the first and second toes, and surgery. Surgery requires straightening the big toe and removal of the bunion. Severe angulation at the metatarsophalangeal joint can cause wearing away of the joint and result in arthritis in that joint. In severe cases, surgery is more beneficial earlier than later.

## HAMMER TOE

*Hammer Toes* are a contracture of the middle joint on the toes. Variations occur with contracture of the distal joint in the toes. If the toes are flexible enough to be manipulated straight, a hammer toe pad can be used to keep them straight. Frequently, calluses will form over the top of the bent portion of the hammer toes, causing pain and inflammation. Surgery may be performed if this condition cannot be treated conservatively.

## FRACTURES IN THE FOOT

Fractures may occur to any bone in the foot and should always be ruled out with an x-ray whenever there has been trauma to the foot.

Fractures in the toes frequently are treated with taping unless a joint is involved. Other fractures in the foot may be treated with casting or, in severe fractures, with surgery.

## STRESS FRACTURES

Stress fractures are frequently found in the foot. Excessive, repeated loading of the bones in the foot may cause a stress fracture although in about half the cases, x-rays fail to show it. If there is suspicion of a stress fracture, a bone scan with radio isotopes can confirm the diagnosis.

When a stress fracture has been identified, resting the area for four to eight weeks is necessary. Sometimes casting is necessary for two to six weeks. Before resuming the sport, the athlete should be symptom free, which usually takes six to eight weeks.

## INJURY TO THE ANKLE JOINT

The *ankle joint* is made up of three bones: the *talus*, the *tibia* and *fibula*. The two leg bones join to form what is called *ankle mortis*. This mortis is more or less the socket for the ankle bone or the talus, which rotates in a hinge-type fashion. The tibia and fibula are joined together by a thick, strong ligament called a *syndesmosis*. The ankle joint is supported by a joint capsule and by strong medial and lateral ankle ligaments.

There are three distinct strong ligaments on the outside of the ankle which give support to the lateral aspect of the ankle. They restrain the foot and ankle from turning in. Excessive turning in of the ankle (inversion) or excessive supination of the foot causes the classic ankle sprain.

On the inside, the ankle is supported by a very strong ligament called the *deltoid ligament* which protects and restrains the ankle from turning to the outside.

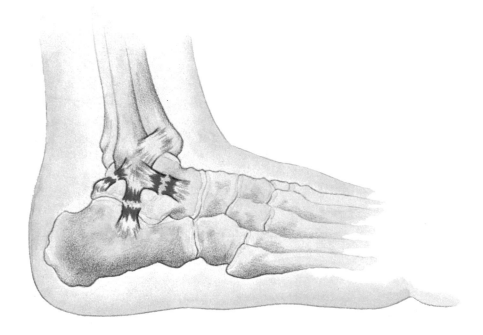

*Diagram of the lateral aspect of the ankle showing a third degree sprain of a complete tear of the lateral ankle ligaments.*

## SPRAINS OF THE ANKLE JOINT

In classic ankle sprain, the ankle turns in too far, tearing the lateral ankle ligaments. This, like other sprains, is graded into first- second- and third- degree. First-degree sprain is characterized by minimal swelling, slight tenderness, and rapid healing. In second-degree sprains, more of the ligaments are torn and stretched and slight instability results. The ankle definitely needs to be supported with an ankle brace or a cast for six weeks. Also, coordination and strength with ankle exercises is emphasized during and after the healing phase. Third-degree ankle sprains involve complete rupture of the ligaments and instability of the ankle. This means that the talus can be completely turned in and rocked out of its joint due to complete rupture of the lateral ligaments. This can be treated with a brace or a cast. Sometimes surgery is necessary to repair the ligaments.

Of the three ankle ligaments, the most commonly injured is the *anterior talofibular ligament*. Injured in about 70% of the cases, this is the ligament in front and on the lateral side of the ankle. The large ligament on the inside of the ankle is called the *deltoid ligament* and only about ten percent of ankle injuries occur from damage to it. When instability results, as in a third-degree sprain of the deltoid ligament, surgery is often necessary.

Severe injuries to the ankle ligaments should always be checked by a professional to make sure there is no instability to the ankle joint and that there is no other injury such as a fracture or spreading of the ankle mortis. If instability or other fractures are found, surgery may be necessary to restore stability to the ankle.

## FRACTURES TO THE ANKLE JOINT

When a fracture to the ankle joint occurs, it is absolutely necessary to restore the ankle joint to its original anatomic position. That is, to put back the pieces exactly where they were. If this is not done, a chronic, painful and unstable ankle joint will result, ending an athletic career or causing a chronic and painful condition in a non-athlete.

# FRACTURE OF THE TALUS

A fracture across the neck of the talus can sometimes cause loss of the blood supply to the part of the talus which is in the ankle joint, causing a **severe** problem to the ankle.

Small chips in the talus are sometimes mistaken for ankle sprains. These are usually not serious unless they are loose inside the ankle joint, and are seen on x-ray as small chips inside the ankle joint. Sometimes surgery is necessary to remove them.

# INJURIES TO THE LOWER LEG

The lower leg is composed of two bones, and the top part of the lower leg forms the plateau for the knee joint. The two bones forming the lower leg are the *tibia* (the larger bone) and the *fibula* (the smaller bone). These two bones come together on the lower end to form the ankle joint.

The muscles in back of the leg, or *calf muscles*, attach to the largest tendon in the body, the *Achilles tendon*. This tendon attaches to the heel bone or the *calcaneus*, giving us the ability to push off on the foot or stand on our tip toes. Muscles in the front part of the leg are located between the tibia and fibula and lie more to the outside of the leg. These muscles attach to long tendons which extend down into the foot, extending or lifting up the toes and lifting up the foot. Other muscles, found in the deep part of the leg behind the tibia underneath the calf muscles, flex the toes. This area also contains the posterior tibial muscle.

The muscles are enclosed in a tight, inflexible compartment of connective tissue or *fascia*. When an injury to the muscle inside these compartments causes swelling, pressure builds inside the compartment, resulting in pain.

If the pressure becomes severe, a *compartment syndrome* can result. This means the pressure is so great that the blood supply to the muscle is compromised. This can cause severe damage and should be recognized and treated immediately. Acute compartment syndromes are usually the result of external direct impact to the soft tissue, causing bleeding or a muscle rupture inside the compartment.

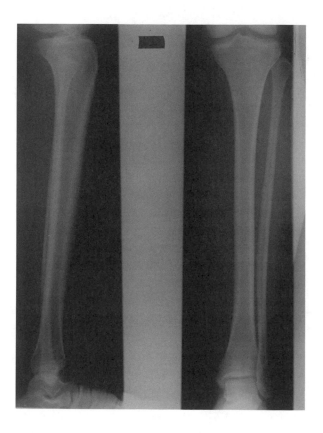

*This is a normal x-ray of the lower leg showing the knee joint and the ankle joint.*

*Subacute compartment syndromes* develop more slowly than acute compartment syndromes. They are caused by many small tears within the muscle, resulting in swelling and increased pressure in the muscle compartment. This is usually a stress or overuse injury, commonly caused by exercising without having properly prepared the body through conditioning and flexibility training.

*Chronic compartment syndromes* build up over a long period of time. They are usually due to enlargement of muscle tissue with prolonged training. When muscle tissue expands to a point where it is larger than the surrounding fascia, the increasing pressure causes pain during exercise. The condition continues to get worse as exercise continues.

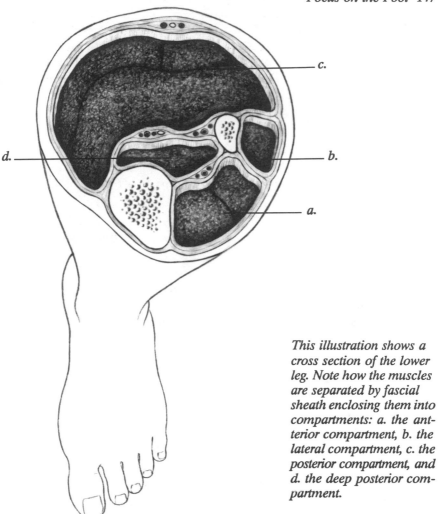

*This illustration shows a cross section of the lower leg. Note how the muscles are separated by fascial sheath enclosing them into compartments: a. the antterior compartment, b. the lateral compartment, c. the posterior compartment, and d. the deep posterior compartment.*

This mechanism is easy to understand. At rest, the enlarged muscle fits snugly into the non-elastic fascia compartment surrounding the muscle. With exercise, the capillaries dilate, blood flow increases and the muscle expands within the tight compartment. This increases pressure, restricting blood flow. When blood flow is restricted and the muscle continues to work, lactic acid is built up. The lactic acid build-up yields more swelling, causing further increase in pressure, and further limitation occurs. If the vicious cycle is allowed to continue, muscle damage can result.

Compartment syndromes can cause pain in the front, back or side of the lower leg and can have sudden or slow onset. Persistent pain or severe pain in the lower leg should be evaluated by an orthopedist. Pressures can be measured within the compartment. If the pressure exceeds a certain level, surgery may be necessary to relieve the pressure and prevent severe and permanent muscle damage. If recognized early, compartment syndromes can be treated non-surgically with elevation, ice, physical therapy and evaluation of the cause. Surgery is only done as a last resort to save the muscle.

Another cause for pain in the lower leg is "shin splints." This is the wastebasket term for pain in the lower leg. Actual causes of shin splints usually include inflammation of the tendon sheath, inflammation of the muscle or tendon attachments to the bone or compartment syndrome. When this pain persists, tibial stress fractures must always be considered.

Normally, shin splints last a few days after beginning a new exercise and will resolve with stretching, icing and anti-inflammatory medication. Persistence of this kind of pain should always be evaluated by a health professional.

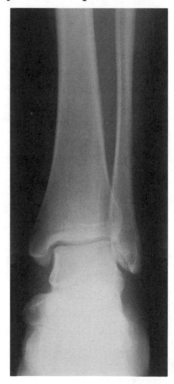

*A stress fracture of the fibula due to repeated loading during running.*

# STRESS FRACTURES OF THE TIBIA AND FIBULA

The tibia or fibula are not uncommon places for stress fractures to occur due to prolonged and repeated loading, such as in distance running or repeated jumping.

## FRACTURES

### FRACTURES IN THE LOWER LEG

Fractures of the bones in the lower leg are very serious, seen frequently in Alpine skiers and players of collision sports such as football, rugby and soccer. Many of us remember watching television and seeing Joe Thiesman, quarterback for the Washington Redskins, fracture both bones of the lower leg while playing football. Fractures of both bones of the lower leg or of either the tibia or fibula alone should always be seen and treated appropriately by a specialist. Sometimes surgery may be required.

### ACHILLES INJURIES

*Achilles tendinitis*, or inflammation of the Achilles tendon, is caused by lack of good flexibility training and stretching of the Achilles tendon, and/or improper warm-ups prior to running. This results in micro tears of the tendon and can lead to a chronic inflammation. Tendinitis can also lead to deterioration and breakdown if the condition becomes chronic.

### RUPTURE OF THE ACHILLES TENDON

Complete rupture of the Achilles tendon occurs suddenly and is felt as a severe, painful "pop" in the back of the calf. Some people say it felt like something exploded in the back of the calf. Afterwards, the athlete cannot walk normally and cannot push off with the foot or stand on tip toes. The area over the Achilles tendon is swollen and tender and shows bruising. A defect can usually be felt in the tendon.

Complete rupture of the Achilles should be surgically repaired. That is, the torn ends should be sutured back together soon after the injury. This is followed by cast immobilzation and bracing. Full strength and motion are regained slowly over months of physical therapy.

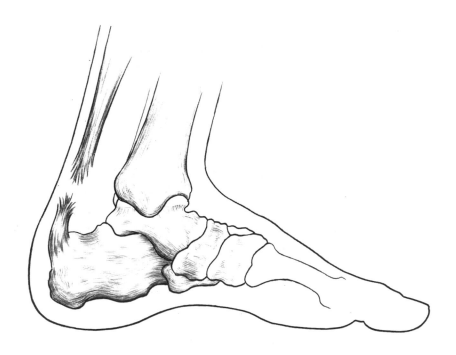

*A complete rupture of the Achilles tendon.*

As you might have guessed by now, many recreational athletes have a tendency to overdo things. When they get into basketball, tennis or running, they'll go too hard, too soon, too often. A nice way to stay healthy is to make use of the word "too" and divide everything you aren't physically prepared to do by it. For example, if you haven't played tennis for awhile, and you usually play for two hours...play for one. If you normally walk for 40 to 60 minutes, but have been inactive for a couple of weeks, you got it, 20 to 30 minutes max. I guarantee that afterwards you'll feel less fatigued, less stressed ....and DEFINITELY less injured.

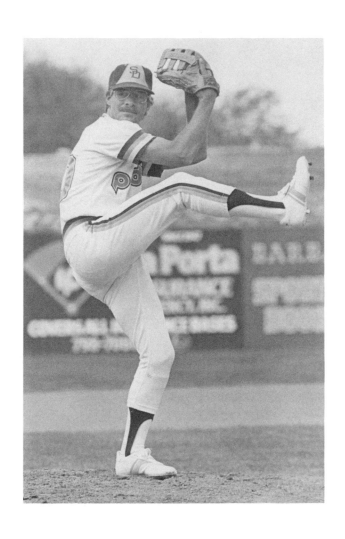

**Chapter Nine**
# Upper Extremity

# Upper Extremity

What's that you say, Bunky? When you get out of bed in the morning your shoulders ache so bad you find yourself identifying with the large "No Shoulder" and "Shoulder Under Repair" signs on the highway? Well, you're not alone. Shoulder, elbow and wrist injuries are about as common nowadays as roads under repair.

## THE UPPER EXTREMITY

The upper extremity, when functioning normally, is a marvel of motion and integration of muscular activity. The complex known as the shoulder girdle has the greatest mobility of all the joints of the body. The majority of the motion is attained because of a ball-in-socket type joint in the shoulder girdle. While the elbow is highly versatile, it is a smoothly functioning hinge-type joint between the precisely-fitted bone endings of the lower and upper arm. The hinge type of joint allows less motion, but is more stable.

The arm and shoulder are involved in the most routine movements. Man uses his arms and shoulders more than any other portion of the body. Even while breathing, there is a slight movement of the shoulder socket-joint where it meets the upper arm.

## THE SHOULDER

Most of us think of the shoulder joint as being one joint, where the upper arm meets the collar bone. Not so. There are four joints that form the shoulder complex, and this composite of four joints must move in harmony, by muscle action, for perfect efficiency of motion. Each joint is dependent upon the others, and any problem in one joint affects them all. The shoulder socket is a part of the *scapula* (shoulder blade). The upper arm bone (*humerus*) fits into this socket, forming the *glenohumeral joint*. In the front, the scapula attaches to the breastbone by way of the collar bone (*clavicle*), forming the *acromioclavicular joint*. The collarbone attaches to the breastbone at the *sternoclavicular joint*. In the back, the scapula is held to the back chest wall by muscles which are called the *scapulothoracic joint*. Although this is not a true joint, approximately one-third of the shoulder motion comes from here.

As the arm goes through its wide range of motion, there is literally a symphony of muscular action unfolding. As certain muscles contract to raise the arm, other muscles must relax at precisely the correct time to allow freedom of motion and smoothness of movement. There are over 20 muscles directly or indirectly involved in shoulder action, needing complex integration of muscle activity (coordination).

The bones themselves are rigid, but movement of the arm and shoulder becomes possible where two bones join. You should be able to rotate your arm painlessly through an angle of 180 degrees. If your shoulder joint is normal, you can make a complete circle at the shoulder with your arm, as well as an infinite number of other complex manipulations.

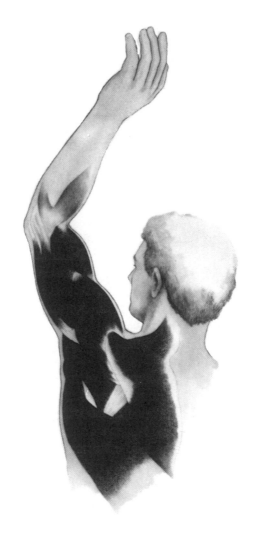

*Complex integration of muscle and nerve activity is needed to raise the arm over the head.*

The versatility of your upper limbs is due to a series of splendid joints in the fingers, wrists, elbows and shoulders which allow the arm to twist, turn and bend. Bone, muscle, tendon, ligament and nerve must work together in an intimate relationship to move the arm and shoulder with precision. Bones give the arm its tensile strength, while the limb is moved by skeletal muscles which may be attached directly to the bone or through connecting tendons. Ligaments prevent the bones from slipping apart at the joints.

Painless, carefree movement in the arm and shoulder (as well as in most other joints) is possible because portions of the bones, where they meet, are lined with a smooth layer of cartilage. In addition, freely movable joints are held together by a capsule of connective tissue called a *synovial capsule*. The lining of the synovial capsule secretes a fluid which allows the bones of the arm and shoulder to slide easily and painlessly against one another at the joints.

Because the shoulder has so many joints and movable parts, it is often involved in sports injuries. The ball-and-socket of the shoulder, for example, is the most easily dislocated of all the joints, and the shoulder girdle is one of the most intricate systems of joints.

## SHOULDER PAIN

The three basic elements of the arm and shoulder (the bone, muscle and joint tissue) act in perfect rhythm, provided the nerves are functioning normally. When nerves are impinged by injury to the shoulder, there is usually pain and abnormal limits of motion.

Shoulder pain does not always come from the actual shoulder joint or joints. It may come from another area of the body, but is felt in the shoulder as pain. This is called *referred pain*, and can be due to compressed nerves in the neck, upper back, chest or arm. Pain can also come from muscle origin in the neck or chest. Heart pain is sometimes felt in the shoulder. Pain may also come from bone in the shoulder complex.

Pain in the joint itself is frequently caused by irritation or inflammation of the joint lining (synovium). The cartilage surface may become worn out, causing degenerative arthritis. Tendons are also a frequent source of pain such as *biceps tendinitis* or *rotator cuff tendinitis*.

Many persons complaining of arm and shoulder pain have a condition called *bursitis* arising from the bursa. A *bursa* is the synovial pouch which secretes a lubricating *synovial fluid* that tendons, muscle and bone need in order to slide over each other. When a bursa becomes irritated, inflamed and swollen, it can be very painful to move the affected area.

Often arthritis, tendinitis or bursitis is secondary to another primary problem. Inflammation develops as a result of some irritating factor. A shoulder which is not moving in a synchronous manner becomes irritated, resulting in inflammation. **The synchronous movement of the shoulder joint is absolutely dependent upon coordinated activity of all the muscles involved in shoulder activity.**

When the diagnosis of arthritis or bursitis is made, anti-inflammatory medication is often administered, either in tablet form or by injection directly into the shoulder structure. These medications offer much-needed relief, but knowing the cause of the inflammation is essential. In this way, not only the symptom but the cause can be treated. Any time arthritis or bursitis is present in a shoulder, the muscular strength and coordination of all the muscles involved with shoulder activity must be examined.

When an area is inflamed and painful, the body responds by shutting down the muscle, thereby limiting the ROM (Range of Motion) of the area involved. The body will also avoid that muscle and use another muscle to move that region of the body. This is called *muscle substitution*. The joint will move, but not correctly or efficiently, possibly causing further damage and inflammation. This can happen in any joint of the body, but is especially important to consider in the shoulder since the shoulder is so dependent upon proper control.

A severe tendinitis which is very painful can cause a frozen shoulder because of lack of movement of the glenohumeral joint. Because approximately one-third of the shoulder's motion can still be accomplished through the other joints in the shoulder complex, the lack of movement in the glenohumeral joint may be neglected, allowing scar tissue to form. If not treated early, it may be difficult to regain total motion. A mild tendinitis may cause no loss of motion, but continued use of this shoulder can result in further inflammation and eventually, small tears of the tendon. Constant irritation over a period of time may cause severe tendon problems.

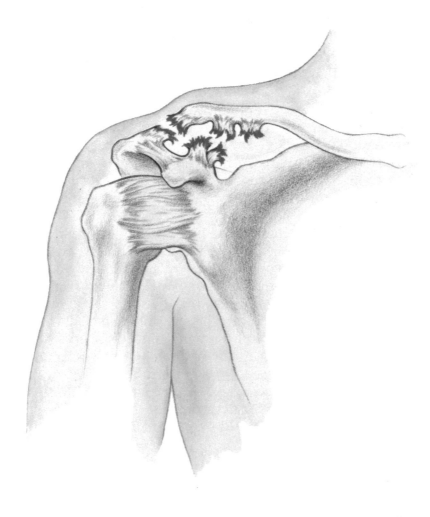

*A third degree AC separation showing the clavicle separated from the acromion. The ligaments holding down the clavicle have been torn.*

## ACROMIOCLAVICULAR SPRAIN
### "AC Separation"

The joint between the collar bone and the shoulder blade is often injured in contact sports events. This injury is usually caused by a direct blow to the top of the shoulder, as when the athlete hits the ground hard. This is called an "*AC separation.*" (Although, technically, it is a sprain, because the ligaments have been torn.) It can be mild or severe and may require immobilization or surgery, depending upon whether it is a first-degree, second-degree or third-degree separation or sprain.

## THE SHOULDER SOCKET

The ligaments hold bone to bone much like straps or ropes, and they are a component of all joints. The glenohumeral joint of the shoulder is a ball-and-socket joint commonly called "the shoulder joint." It is the most mobile joint of the body.

Look at the anatomy of the shoulder. You see a large ball in a small socket, which gives the shoulder its extensive mobility or range of motion. Only 25% of the surface of the *humerus* (the ball) is in contact with the *glenoid fossa* (the socket). As you look at the bony stability of the joint, you can readily see there must be something holding the joint in place. This job is done by ligaments and a joint capsule.

This capsule attaches to a thickened piece of cartilage called *labrum* that surrounds the articular surface of the cavity (joint surface), adding stability. When a dislocation of the shoulder joint occurs, the ball completely slips out of the socket, and the ligamentous structure around the shoulder tears.

## THE DISLOCATED SHOULDER

When the shoulder dislocates, the capsule or labrum tears off the bony rim of the glenoid. The problem here is that once the dislocation has occurred, the tear of the capsule, or the labium, may not heal. If a tear does not heal in proper position, the shoulder will continue to dislocate or partially dislocate. The term used to describe this condition of partial dislocation is *sublux.* When it happens again, it is called recurrent dislocation or *recurrent subluxation* of the shoulder.

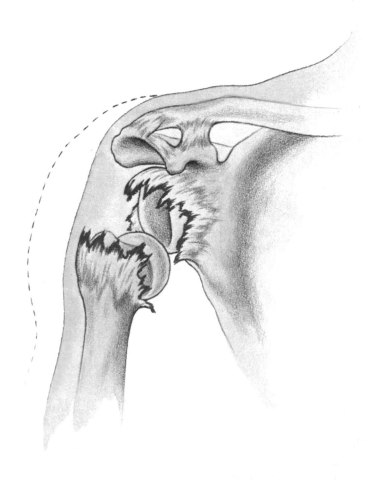

*Diagram of shoulder dislocation. When a shoulder dislocates, the ball completely slips out of the socket, tearing the restraining structures around the joint.*

There are many factors that determine whether or not, after the first dislocation, the shoulder will have a recurring dislocation. Some of these factors are: the amount of trauma in the initial injury, the age of the patient, and the treatment that follows the injury. After a first-time dislocation, the most important remedy is to reduce the dislocation as soon as possible. Only a qualified physician should attempt this. Always have the shoulder checked by a qualified physician at a medical care facility. X-rays should be taken to insure that it is indeed a dislocation. It could be some other injury--such as a fracture which, if treated as a dislocation, could result in severe problems.

After the *reduction* (putting the shoulder back in place), the shoulder should be immobilized (held in place) close to the body with a sling for four to six weeks. This treatment offers the best chance for healing and avoiding a recurrent dislocation.

If, after the first dislocation, the shoulder dislocates again, there is very little chance that it will heal by additional immobilization in a sling. The best way to handle a recurrent dislocation is to undergo surgery to repair ligaments in the shoulder. Surgery will tighten the shoulder joint and prevent further dislocation. Surgery to reconstruct ligaments of the shoulder can now be done using new techniques in arthroscopic surgery.

Subluxation of the shoulder means that the shoulder is not completely out of the joint. It is an unstable shoulder joint; the ball or the humerus slides forward, then backward in the glenoid of the socket. It is a common occurrence when the arm goes into an external rotation and an abducted position (in other words, a throwing position). Symptoms may be pain in the shoulder or a "dead" arm feeling. It actually feels as if the arm has partially slipped out of the joint.

Treatment of this condition involves certain exercises for the shoulder. Since the shoulder is such a dynamic joint, meaning that a good deal of the stability of the joint comes from surrounding muscles, some of the symptoms of a slightly unstable joint improve if the muscles are working together properly. This requires strength and coordination. If physical therapy or therapeutic exercise is unsuccessful, a surgical approach is necessary. Surgery is often effective and satisfying to the patient.

Tears of the glenoid labrum can have symptoms similar to those of recurrent subluxation. Often these may be part of a subluxation or dislocation problem. Arthroscopic surgery may again be the answer for this injury.

## THE ROTATOR CUFF

Rotator cuff injuries require a little more explanation. Two thirds of the motion in the shoulder comes from the glenohumeral joint, the ball-and-socket part of the shoulder. The motion or rotation of the glenohumeral joint is accomplished by the *rotator cuff*, the tendinous attachment of the muscles to the humerus or the ball.

As these muscles contract and relax together, the shoulder rotates. The muscles are solidly attached, or originate from the shoulder blade and attach onto the humerus. For example, the outward rotation of the shoulder is simply the contraction of the *infraspinatus* and *teres muscles* and relaxation of the *subscapularis muscle* or the muscles in front of the shoulder blade. With this synergistic (working together) action, the ball and socket joint moves inward and outward. It is a symphony of partial relaxations and contractions that happens very quickly and allows rotation of the shoulder.

The supraspinatus tendon attaches to the supraspinatus muscle and, when it contracts, it pulls and lifts the arm upward and outward from the body. The unique feature of the supraspinatus (or the part of the rotator cuff which is on top of the joint), is that it injures frequently. Why? Because of its precarious or vulnerable position underneath the acromion process of the shoulder just on top of the ball.

When the ball rotates underneath the acromion process, the rotator cuff can become pinched, causing an *impingement syndrome*. Inflammation of the rotator cuff results from the mechanical irritation of the tendons of the rotator cuff by the impingement (pinching), causing rotator cuff tendinitis or supraspinatus tendinitis.

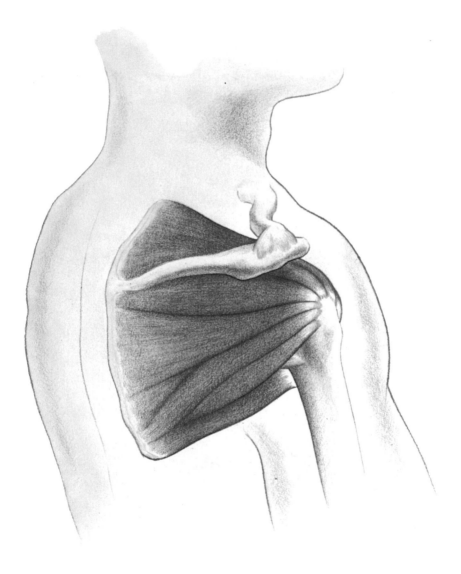

*The rotator cuff muscles surround the humerus. Contraction of
these muscles rotates the ball in the socket. Deltoid muscle,
which overlies the rotator cuff, is not shown.*

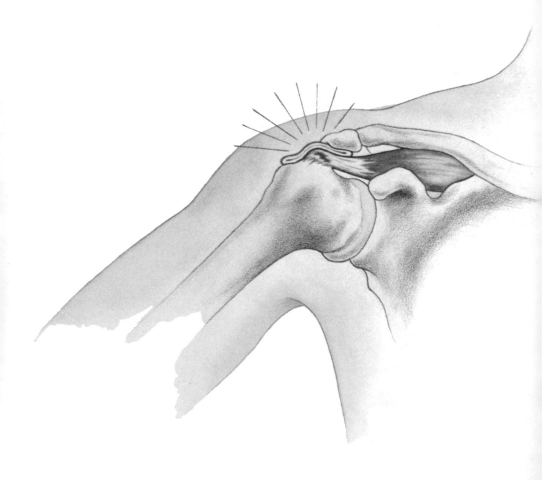

*Impingement syndrome. This illustrates the pinching of the rotator cuff tendon by the under surface of the acromion process.*

This impingement traps tissue between the head of the humerus, acromion process and coraco-acromial ligament. The impingement is most pronounced during arm movement, forward and upward. When it rotates internally in this position, it causes a pinching of the tissues in the anterior parts of the shoulder. This is a common injury in swimmers or any athlete who has forward shoulder posture.

With improper posture, with the scapula rotated forward, the anterior portion of the acromion process is forward and can easily impinge when the arm lifts upward. With proper posture, the shoulder blade is in position to allow the arm to move forward and up, without bumping against the under-surface of the acromion. Frequently, treatment for a mild impingement syndrome is, first, to improve shoulder postural coordination. You can prevent this condition with proper postural coordination of the shoulder at an early age. Untreated impingement syndrome can lead to a tear of the rotator cuff.

The subacromial bursa, which overlies the supraspinatus tendon, helps the supraspinatus tendon glide underneath the acromion process. This rubbing of the supraspinatus tendon, which is an impingement of the tendon under the acromion process, also irritates the bursa overlying the tendon (*See diagram.*) When the bursal sac becomes inflamed, it is called *subacromial bursitis.* In subacromial bursitis, the bursa itself sometimes becomes so painful and swollen that the patient is unable to move the arm.

Often the patient enters the emergency room with excruciating pain. Injections into the bursa are frequently given to relieve the pressure and inflammation. However, treatment should not end here. The underlying cause of the bursitis should be identified and treated, sometimes with physical therapy.

In more severe cases, recurrence of this pinching over a long period of time can cause decreased blood supply to the tendinous area. This, in turn, can cause more inflammation and a breakdown of the tendon, resulting in a ruptured tendon or a *rotator cuff tear.* This happens frequently with older patients, after a number of years of impingement syndrome. The weakest point of the supraspinatus tendon is at a point about a half inch from its insertion or attachment.

A complete rupture of the rotator cuff tendon renders the athlete helpless to lift the arm. When the muscle is no longer attached to the bone, it is nearly impossible to lift the shoulder. Sometimes muscle substitution, such as using the shoulder blade, can fool the patient into thinking that movement is still present. It is not. Meanwhile, the shoulder becomes more contracted, harder to move, and more difficult to treat.

Treatment for complete rupture of the rotator cuff is surgical. Arthroscopic surgery of partial tears of the rotator cuff is frequently successful. Complete tears of the rotator cuff most commonly need surgical repair, followed by physical therapy.

## THE ELBOW

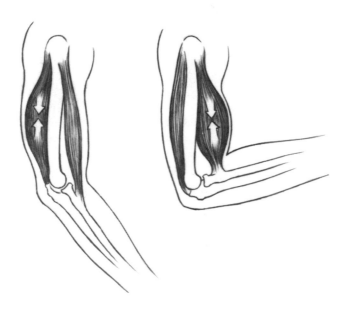

*This illustration of the elbow joint shows the ligamentous structures laterally. The biceps muscle with its tendon attachment to the radius contracts and flexes the elbow. The triceps and triceps tendon attachment posterially contracts and extends the elbow.*

The elbow joint is a hinge joint that allows flexion and extension of the forearm on the upper arm with contraction of the biceps and triceps muscles. This means that shortening contractions of the biceps, combined with lengthening or relaxation of the triceps, gives flexion of the elbow, and vice-versa for extension or straightening of the elbow. When the forearm moves from palm up (supination) to palm down (pronation), motion must occur in both the elbow and wrist by the two forearm bones—the *radius* and the *ulna*. This action comes from rotation of the radius bone around the ulna at the wrist. At the wrist, with the supination/pronation movement, the radius rotates in a "radius" around the stationary ulna. The ulna, fastened to the end of the arm, secures itself in the *olecranon fossa*. The *radial head* is the end of the radius at the elbow joint; it is round and disc-shaped to allow rotation of the forearm at the elbow.

The muscles of the forearm that flex and extend the wrist are anchored to the bony prominences of the elbow called the medial and lateral *epicondyle*. The medial side of the elbow is the side next to the body with the arms down in a palm up position. The lateral epicondyle is on the outside.

Inflammation can occur, secondary to micro tears, where the tendons of the forearm muscles are anchored to the epicondyles. This is called *epicondylitis*. Medial epicondylitis is commonly seen in throwing sports or in sports using more wrist flexion. Stress occurs across the medial aspect of the elbow when the wrist goes into flexion, pulling on the muscle attachment. This repeated stress may cause micro tears and inflammation around the epicondyle.

Inflammation of the outside of the elbow is called *lateral epicondylitis*. This is due to the contraction of the wrist extensors. Athletes who are using the wrist extensor muscles, such as with the backhand movement that tennis players are fond of, often get "tennis elbow." Again, this is an inflammation of the tendon where it attaches to the bone.

## TENNIS ELBOW

Symptoms of "tennis elbow" are pain at the elbow and secondary weakness of the wrist extension. Tennis elbow (lateral epicondylitis) strikes players of tennis, badminton, table tennis and golf. Frequently this is caused by a faulty backhand—using too much wrist—or using the wrong size racquet. It also happens as a non-sport injury to workers such as electricians and carpenters.

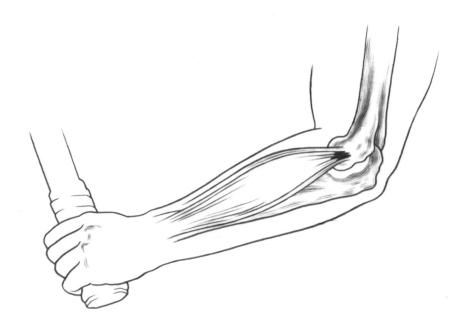

*"Tennis elbow," or lateral epicondylitis, is inflammation or tearing of the tendon attachment of the wrist extensor muscles at the elbow.*

Lateral epicondylitis can be caused by any motion that uses frequent extension of the wrist. Likewise, faulty forehand technique can cause inflammation of the medial epicondyle. Abnormal stress across this lateral epicondyle may cause inflammation or small tears of the tendon. Although it is more common in athletes over forty, the incidence of tennis elbow in those who play is up to 45%.

# THROWING MOTION

This is a complex movement that has four parts. They are: wind-up, cocking, acceleration, and deceleration or follow-through. Throwing injuries most frequently affect the shoulder and the elbow. Injury to the shoulder and elbow are not common in the wind-up stage, but much stress moves across the anterior shoulder and the medial aspect of the elbow in the cocking stage.

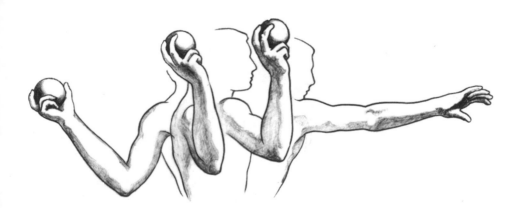

*The complex throwing motion.*

During this stage, the shoulder is at the abducted, externally-rotated position, or rather a hyper-extended externally rotated position. The elbow is flexed at about 45 degrees. The forward motion then begins, starting the third stage acceleration. At that point the stress starts across the front of the shoulder and medial aspect of the elbow.

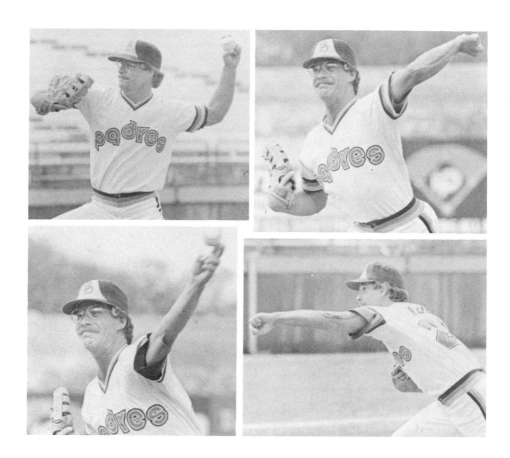

*Stages of throwing motion: wind-up (not shown), cocking,
acceleration (2 phases), deceleration.*

The acceleration or forward motion stage is composed
of two parts, beginning with bringing the arm forward with the
wrist cocked. In this extended position, there is more stress
across the medial aspect of the elbow and some compression
across the lateral aspect of the elbow. This is followed by the
second phase of acceleration, in which the shoulder rapidly
rotates inward and the hand and forearm are snapped forward.
This is the phase that may cause injury to the growth plate in
young athletes. The fourth stage of the throwing motion, deceleration or follow through, starts at ball release, characterized by the forearm going into pronation.

Frequent injuries resulting from the throwing motion are: rotator cuff tendinitis, biceps tendinitis, elbow or medial epicondylitis, and triceps tendinitis at the elbow.

Injury to the ulnar nerve often happens to throwers. The ulnar nerve lies along the medial aspect of the elbow. With the stresses in the cocking position of the first phase of acceleration, the nerve may stretch and become irritated. This can cause numbness in the little finger or the ring finger and sometimes necessitates surgical treatment.

## "LITTLE LEAGUE ELBOW"

Throwing injuries in the young athlete, commonly called "Little League Elbow," can be serious. This may develop from a heavy pitching schedule. Although a Little Leaguer, by rule, can only pitch up to six innings per week, this only limits the number of throws he makes in competition as a pitcher. It does not limit the amount of hard throws he may pitch in practice, nor does the rule prohibit the same pitcher throwing the ball as a part-time catcher. **This is important to monitor.** Studies have shown that injuries to the elbow in young athletes 9 to 14 years old are directly proportional to the number of throws executed.

Another factor in the injury rate of these young athletes is whether or not the child throws curve balls. If he does, he stands a higher risk of developing an injury. Between 12 and 20% of young pitchers have physical problems related to throwing.

During the acceleration phase, the thrower's arm pulls forward with the forearm lagging, putting much stress across the elbow. Problems in the medial side of the elbow are caused by pulling forces (distraction forces) called *valgus stress*. X-rays of the elbow may show changes in the growing cartilage and bone (the medial growth plate) of the young athlete. The more severe problems, however, are on the lateral side, where repeated jamming or compression of the cartilage surface of the radius bone (radial head) against the *capitulum* (the upper portion of the elbow joint) may cause loss of blood to the radial head. When this occurs, loose pieces of cartilage and bone are often left in the joint, leading to arthritis. About eight percent of younger pitchers had elbow x-ray changes showing some damage to the lateral side of the elbow.

It is not uncommon to see loose pieces of cartilage, called *loose bodies*, in the elbows of teenagers who were pitchers at a younger age. Surgery is often necessary to remove the loose pieces in the elbow if the symptoms are pain, "locking" of the elbow and lack of full motion. Sometimes this can be done arthroscopically.

Good throwing mechanics and pre-game warm-up, combined with good shoulder coordination and not throwing with "all arm" would help prevent elbow problems in young athletes. Proper certification before coaching or training young players is one proposed approach. Education in injury prevention for Little League coaches, parents and players would reduce the injury rate as well. Certainly a teamwork of education and communication between coaches, trainers, parents and players, through whatever effective means available, is definitely needed to reduce injury rates. Young players should be educated and encouraged to report any type of soreness that may arise. There should be icing of the elbow following practice and play and decreased amounts of throwing altogether (such as missing rotations, not throwing in practice or not moving from pitcher to catcher's positions). All of this would help spare the arm of the Little League pitcher.

If symptoms of injury persist with the young athlete, x-rays should be taken and the Little Leaguer checked by a specialist. Abnormal stress put on growing, immature tissues can cause lifelong problems.

## NERVE ENTRAPMENTS

Pain in the elbow can be caused by nerve entrapments. Nerve entrapments of the medial, radial or ulnar nerves at the elbow are frequent causes of problems in the elbow. If these become severe, weakness and numbness result, and surgery may be required.

## DISLOCATION OF THE ELBOW

One of the more severe injuries is a dislocation of the elbow, perhaps accompanied by a fracture dislocation. This should be seen by a qualified orthopedic surgeon as soon as possible. Sometimes surgery is necessary to reduce the fracture. There should be testing to make sure there are no ligament tears, and x-rays should be taken to assure proper position of the bones at the elbow. If improperly treated, the dislocated elbow may result in a contracture of the elbow. That is, the elbow may never regain full motion. Fractures about the elbow are serious, especially in children. They can cause growth disturbances and even vascular compromise. In turn, this can cause a permanent injury to the forearm in a child.

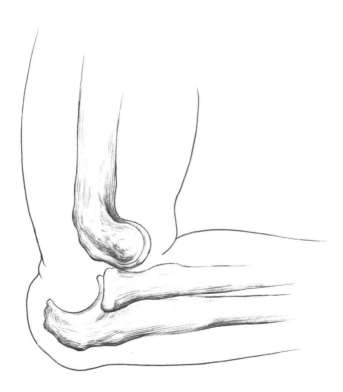

*Dislocation of the elbow joint.*

## WRIST INJURIES

Wrist injuries such as tendinitis around the wrist are common in athletes and are best treated like tendinitis in other locations. First, decrease the inflammation with rest (possible splinting), anti-inflammatory medication and ice. Then, identify the cause of the problem. Frequently it is caused by weak muscles in the forearm or shoulder, which can be treated with physical therapy.

## FRACTURES OF THE FOREARM

Fractures of both bones in the forearm are very serious and may require surgery to prevent permanent deformity and restriction of forearm motion.

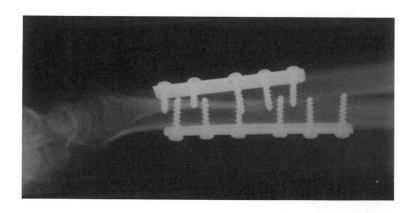

*X-ray of the forearm following surgery after open reduction, internal fixation using metal plates. Note that the bones have been restored to their anatomical position.*

## FRACTURES OF THE WRIST

Fractures of the radius bone at the wrist or fractures of both the radius and ulnar bones are commonly seen as a result of a fall on an outstretched hand. These fractures vary in severity, and treatment varies according to the type and severity of the fracture. Fracture of the distal radius is very common in children.

Another fracture commonly seen after a fall on an outstretched hand is a *navicular fracture*. The navicular bone is one of the small bones in the wrist called the *carpal* bones. This fracture is sometimes passed off as a "wrist sprain," because there is no obvious deformity of the wrist. **This is a mistake.** X-rays should be taken to make sure no fractures are present. If a fracture of the navicular bone is missed and not treated properly, serious problems in the wrist can result.

## INJURIES ABOUT THE WRIST

Other injuries about the wrist include entrapment of the nerves at the wrist level. Entrapment of the median nerve, where it snakes through the carpal tunnel, is very important to recognize, as well as when there is entrapment of the ulnar nerve at the wrist. The median nerve gives sensation to the thumb, index and long fingers. If the nerve is compressed in the carpal tunnel at the wrist, it will cause decreased feeling in these fingers and thumb. They will feel as if they are asleep. This is called *carpal tunnel syndrome* and in more severe cases can cause weakness in the hand. Pinching of the ulnar nerve is less common and causes numbness in the little and ring fingers.

Deep lacerations in the wrist or hand should be checked thoroughly by a qualified physician. Cut nerves or tendons require immediate attention by a surgeon.

## HAND INJURIES

Hand injuries frequently include injuries of the fingers and the finger joints. These injuries are common in contact sports. Often the ball or another player strikes the tips of the fingers, causing a fracture, tearing of the ligaments, or dislocation of the joints. Injuries to the small joints of the fingers can cause tears to the ligaments and instability of the joints. If no instability is found, most of the time treatment is done with "*buddy taping*" (taping the injured finger to a non-injured one) for two to four weeks. This gives a splinting effect but allows motion of the joint. These small joints may stay swollen for some weeks following the injury.

Injury to the tendon attachment of the distal joint of a finger, called a *mallet finger*, happens when the tendon attachment is completely off—either pulled off with a piece of bone or severed. This is common when the fingertip is hit with a ball when the finger is in the extended or straight position.

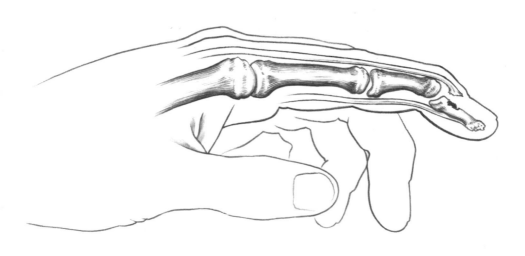

*Mallet finger deformity. A small avulsion of the attachment of the extensor tendon. Without this attachment, the finger will no longer extend.*

When this happens, the distal phalanx will not extend. The flexor tendon attached on the undersurface of the finger keeps it pulled into a mallet-shaped position. Since there is no attachment on the dorsal surface, the finger cannot be straightened or extended. This requires treatment, either placing the finger in a brace, immobilizing splint for up to six weeks, or with surgery. Without treatment, a mallet finger will become a permanently fixed distal joint—a joint that cannot be actively straightened.

Finger dislocations are frequently seen on the sideline at football and basketball events. Coaches and trainers work with finger dislocations all the time without the benefit of an x-ray. Some of these fingers are reduced with no problem and without medical treatment—*unfortunately*, not all of them. If a finger has been dislocated and reduced by the trainer or coach on the field, or even by the sideline physician, follow-up x-rays are still needed. These x-rays will determine if there is a fracture, joint damage or ligament laxity.

Some dislocations occur at the *metacarpophalangeal joint* (where the big knuckles join). These are sometimes called *complex dislocations*. A dislocation at this level is like a Chinese finger trap. It cannot be reduced by simply pulling. The harder the pull, the tighter it gets. This is a complex anatomical problem that requires treatment by a hand specialist who has the ability to unlock this condition. Pulling is *not* the treatment.

### INJURIES TO THE THUMB

Thumb injuries are a common upper extremity sports injury, which often occur while skiing. A condition known as "skier's thumb" is a tear of the ulnar collateral ligament at the base of the *proximalphalanx* (big knuckle) of the thumb. Another term for this is "gamekeeper's thumb," because English gamekeepers used to snap the heads off of small game and, in doing so, they often chronically stretched out the ulnar collateral ligament of their thumbs. This ligament is essential for the stability of a pinch. If this ligament is not functional, due to a complete tear or a third-degree sprain, the effectiveness of the pinching movement is noticeably reduced.

Skiing professionals estimate that up to 200,000 of these thumb injuries occur each year in the U.S. alone. About 10% of skiing injuries involve this area of the thumb, making it the second most common injury in skiing—knee injuries being first. "Skier's thumb" occurs when the skier falls with his thumb outstretched, catching it in the snow, possibly with the pole still in hand.

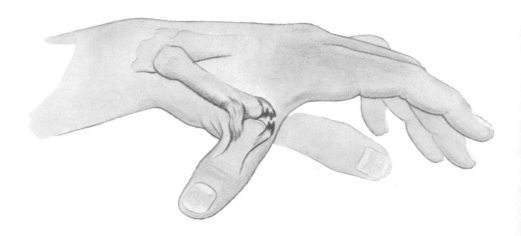

*The ulnar collateral ligaments are completely torn when the thumb is forced out of joint as shown here.*

Although newer, strapless ski poles have not significantly reduced the number of occurrences of this type of thumb injury, other complications to the upper part of the body which result from using straps on ski poles have been affected. (An example would be injuring your shoulder when the strap gets caught in a bush or a tree.) Strapless poles are now thought to be safer.

When a complete tear of the ligament does occur, the torn ligament is frequently trapped underneath another tendon. In order to properly treat this condition, surgery is necessary to free the ligament and sew it together. An evaluation should always be given by a specialist using special x-rays to determine the extent of the injury.

Partial tears of the ulnar collateral ligament can easily be treated in a cast. Complete tears may require surgery. Surgical results of treatment of these tears is very good, whereas the non-surgical treatment can cause instability of the joint, such as the gamekeeper's injury where the stability of the pinch motion is gone. If improperly treated, when a person tries to pick up an object, there is little or no stability in the thumb movement. It can actually sublux out of place. This can be a significant disability.

From the thumb to the shoulder, there is one constant in the world of fitness: injuries happen and they are definitely no fun. But with a little common sense and some proper precautions, you should be able to stay relatively injury—and highway sign—free. Remember to listen and heed the warnings of your body when a shoulder or elbow pain reminds you that it's time to back off....because no one enjoys lifting weights, skiing, throwing a baseball, or playing tennis on a fitness highway constantly under repair.

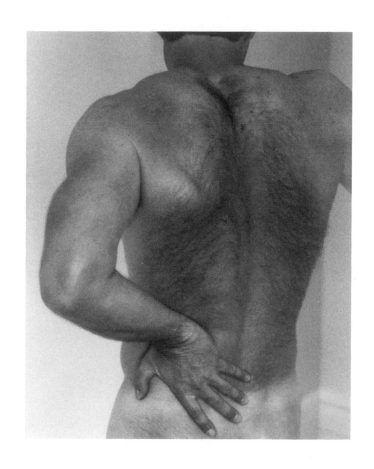

**Chapter Ten**
# The Spine

## Chapter Ten
# The Spine

Let's say that James Bond, good ol' 007 himself, comes to your town to track down that sinister bad guy Evel Dude. Since James is the best of the best in the spy biz, there is a good chance that while he's around he'll be doing some serious spine, right? Wrong, espionage fans! While James Bond definitely has a lot of backbone, he makes his living by "spying." And his spine? That's what helps to make him so darn good at what he does.

### SPINE INJURIES

The spine consists of a series of bones (*vertebra*) stacked on top of each other from the neck to the tail bone. The *cervical spine* consists of seven cervical vertebrae in the neck area. There are twelve thoracic vertebrae in the chest area called the *thoracic spine* and there are normally five *lumbar* vertebrae and one *sacral* vertebra (*sacrum*) forming the *lumbosacral spine* in the lower back area. The lower back is connected to the pelvis by way of the sacrum. The *sacrum* is a large, wide bone at the base of the lower back and it is part of the pelvic ring. Finally, just below the sacrum lies the *coccyx vertebra,* which is commonly known as the tailbone. It serves no function in humans.

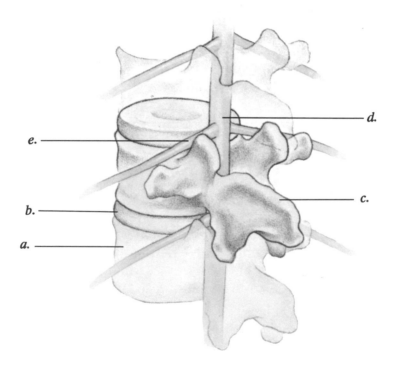

*Diagram of the spinal anatomy showing a. Vertebral body b. Intervertebral disc c. Spinous process d. Spinal chord e. Nerve roots coming off of the spinal chord.*

Each vertebra consists of a vertebral body (anteriorly) and a vertebral arch (posteriorly). The vertebral arch protects the spinal cord while, in front, the vertebral bodies, which give bony stability and height to the spine, are held apart by *intervertebral discs* made of fibrous cartilage. These discs function as shock absorbers and allow movement between the vertebral bodies. The vertebrae, posteriorly, are joined by smaller joints called the *facet joints*, which are held together by complex ligamentous structure and allow movement between each vertebrae. The ligamentous structures, discs, and the bones themselves give the spine its *static* or *passive stability*, the stability provided without muscle support—as when the muscles are relaxed. The *active or dynamic stability* is provided by the muscles of the back.

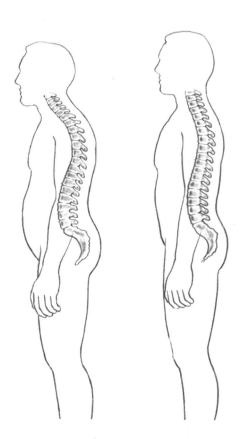

*Poor and Correct Posture*

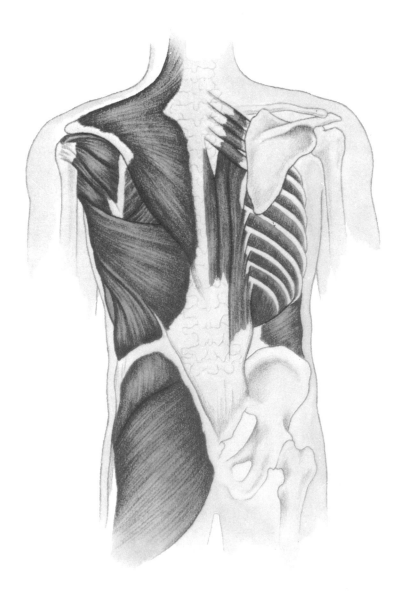

*Diagram of the back showing the muscle attachments and the anatomical relationships.*

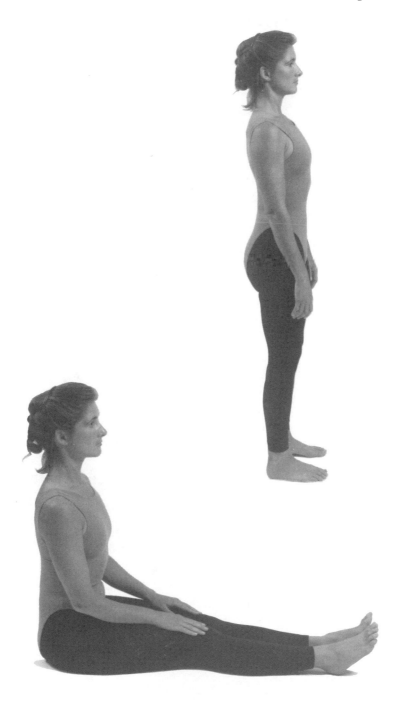

*Examples of good posture*

## POSTURAL COORDINATION

It's important to remember that the muscles in the neck, back, abdomen and rib cage are meant to hold the back in an erect position, balanced against gravity. The action between nerves and muscles that keeps the body erect is called *postural coordination*. Good postural coordination enables the body to move more efficiently, with more agility. It is more than just holding the back straight. It's the entire *carriage* of the body—the position of the shoulders—the position of the hips, knees, ankles and feet when we move. Watch a martial arts expert, or a great dancer. Their posture is excellent. This enables them to use their bodies with great efficiency of movement and to execute complex movements with what seems like little effort.

On the other hand, if you venture out to a local 10k, you'll notice a lot of runners who do not move quite as smoothly as a dancer. Some runners contort their bodies while they run, as if they were getting ready for induction into the Hoola Hoop Hall of Fame.

It is very important to maintain the strength and coordination of the trunk muscles, because when these muscles are weak or the postural coordination is poor, injuries to the discs or the ligaments are common. This is a significant cause of loss of work in industry. In fact, it has been reported that 80% of the population will have some back problem during their lifetimes.

Back complaints are also a common sports-related problem, and one of the main causes for the older beginning athlete to quit exercising. Most of these problems could be prevented by following an exercise program to improve both the strength in the trunk muscles and postural coordination. This is a commonly neglected area in achieving fitness, yet one of the most important to any athlete. **Postural strength and coordination is essential for both injury prevention and sports performance.**

## BACK INJURIES

The most frequently reported back injuries are *lumbar* or lower back strains and sprains. When these occur, it means that there has been too much force across the ligament, which in turn causes swelling and pain. The muscles in the back then reflexively become tight, trying to keep the back from moving more and further injuring the ligaments. This is called *protective spasm*. Normally, these back injuries are treated with rest and anti-inflammatory medication, and sometimes ice. More serious sprains need to be treated with sophisticated physical therapy techniques as well.

Most often, back pain starts as a mild irritation and a nagging ache usually brought on by improper lifting. This ache usually subsides within a few days and is soon forgotten. Until next time! The next experience with back pain will be slightly more painful and will last one to two weeks and may involve time off work and lying flat on your back. This, too, will be forgotten in a short period of time. And yes, you guessed it, there will be a next time! This time the pain will be very severe and a comfortable position will be difficult to find. This bout will surely involve time in bed and probably one to two weeks time off work. This pain can last from one to six months!

These bouts with pain continue, increasing in severity and duration with each episode until the cycle is stopped. Preventing another episode of back pain is more important in this case than actually treating the pain.

## CAUSES OF LOWER BACK PAIN

If the normal soft "S" shaped curve of a healthy back is aligned, the vertebrae absorb stress efficiently with no harmful effects. But poor posture (sitting and standing) combined with the pressure of gravity, adds undue stress to your spine. Over time, the spine will reshape itself in an abnormal position to accommodate this stress, causing a loss or imbalance of the normal spinal curves. This will prohibit normal trunk movement, and cause lower back pain.

Poor flexibility of the legs and hips can also cause lower back pain. This pulls on the pelvis, adding compression to the lumbar spine, throwing your trunk out of balance. Weak abdominal and trunk muscles give the spine no support, forcing the spine itself to take the stress and strain of any movement. These factors are easily corrected with proper physical therapy.

Following the initial evaluation, physical therapy begins with restoring the normal spinal curves through joint mobilization and active therapeutic exercise. Restoring lower extremity flexibility is accomplished through stretching exercises to be followed by an extensive home exercise program to maintain the flexibility gained. Trunk power is accomplished with stabilization and strengthening exercises performed in a consistent and progressive program. Good posture is restored through awareness and education. Often your home or work environment must be adapted slightly to eliminate poor posture and to allow your body to function without any stress factors. Education is crucial. Low back pain patients need to understand which positions and activities are harmful and which are helpful to their back. **Remember, the key to eliminating back pain is in prevention.**

## SCIATICA

Okay, Trivia Fans, it's time for another game of "Stump The Reader."

Sy Atica is:
A) a linebacker for the Green Bay Packers
B) a form of depression that strikes American homeowners when they learn it's time to clean the attic again ("Sy....Atica")
C) a loan shark from New York
D) mispelled. It should be SCIATICA

*Sciatica* is simply pain down the sciatic nerve. The *sciatic nerve* runs down each leg and originates from the combination of nerve roots in the lower back to form the largest nerve in the body, which extends down the buttocks into the back of the thigh. It branches out to give nerve supply to all the muscles in the buttocks and the back of the thigh as well as all the muscles in the lower leg and foot and all the way to the toes. All feeling to the posterior thigh, buttocks and everything below the knee comes by way of the sciatic nerve. Therefore, pressure on one of the nerve roots that joins to form the sciatic nerve can cause pain which is felt all the way down the course of the nerve to the foot. Pain down the nerve (sciatica) can also be caused by direct pressure on the nerve in the buttocks.

Careful examination by a specialist, sometimes followed by sophisticated tests, such as an MRI (Magnetic Resonance Imaging) or nerve conduction studies, can determine where the nerve is being pinched. After this is done, successful treatment can be accomplished, whether it be rest, exercise, physical therapy or surgery. It is important to first find the cause before treatment is initiated.

## STRESS INJURIES AND ARTHRITIS OF THE SPINE

With poor posture and/or weak muscles, the ligaments, bones and joints in the back are constantly taking more of the load than they should because there is little help from the back muscles. This can cause small ligament tears, and breakdown of the intervertebral discs. This in turn, causes pain and muscle spasm. Repetitive stress injury can cause a disc to bulge and weaken, ultimately leading to a ruptured disc and wearing out of the joints themselves (arthritis). Stress fractures occasionally occur in the lower back area. Although they frequently cause pain, they seldom cause paralysis or nerve damage.

Arthritis in the back is not uncommon in the older patient. Repeated wear and tear of the lower back area, due to excess load, results in breakdown (the cartilage in between the joints begins to wear away) and can result in degenerative arthritis of the spine. This, of course, can cause pain and restriction of movement. For this, as well as stress injuries of the back, prevention is the best treatment.

## INJURY TO THE DISCS

Other serious injuries to the back can come in the form of injuries to the *intervertebral disc*. This disc is the fibrocartilage tissue between the body of each vertebra. Structurally, this disc consists of a thick outer portion and a softer central portion. Sometimes it can be injured in a way in which the thick outer portion starts to break down and the inner portion begins to be pushed out. This is similar to a bulge on a tire. Most of the time this is pushed to the back, where the nerve roots exit from the spinal cord on each side.

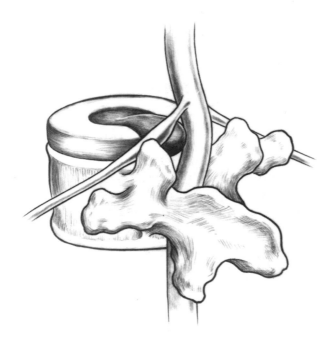

*The diagram illustrates the intervertebral disc bulging and pressing on the nerve root exiting from the spinal canal. This is called a bulging or ruptured disc.*

This bulge can press on the nerve root, causing pain in the back and down the leg (sciatica). A more serious degree of injury to the disc, called a *ruptured disc* or a *herniated disc*, occurs when the center portion of the disc is pushed all the way out and the tough outer portion is completely ruptured. This is similar to the blowout of a tire. The inside portion is completely pushed out onto the spinal cord or the nerve root, causing severe pain and weakness in the legs, in the lower back or both. A herniated or ruptured disc in the neck can cause weakness and pain extending into the shoulder, arm and hand.

Sometimes a ruptured disc can be treated with conservative measures such as rest, proper exercise, and physical therapy. Other times it has to be treated surgically. Professional attention is always necessary.

Susan, a high school teacher with poor postural strength, spends most of her day at her desk and evenings caring for her home and family. She never exercises or does any conditioning because she feels that with all the "running around" she does all day, she has had a full workout before noon. On a day like all the others, she bends over to lift a small stack of books. She suddenly feels a painful snap.

In the course of her everyday activity, she has ruptured a disc in her back and will begin weeks of recovery, possibly including surgery and a physical therapy program. This program will re-educate and strengthen the muscles which, if exercised properly, could have prevented the injury from happening.

This type of injury can happen due to poor muscle strength and postural coordination in the back, and the lack of regular exercise. This causes back muscles to weaken, giving little support to the spinal column. Then, during a normal day's activity, all the load of the body, or too much of the load, is taken up by the ligaments, bones and cartilaginous discs in the back. Something has to give—and it usually does.

There is a happy ending to Susan's story, however, as there is in a growing number of patients recovering from back injuries. Through the course of meetings with her orthopedist and the weeks of physical therapy, she developed an understanding of the importance of proper exercise. And, as a relationship developed between her and her Sports Medicine Team, she discovered that she actually looked forward to the therapy as well as the walking program her doctor prescribed. Susan was hooked. And she became a consistent and loyal Everyday Athlete. Not only was she able to correct the problem, relieve the pain and assist in healing the injury, she took charge of her own body and can now experience the joy that comes from being active and healthy.

Then there's the one about the competitive athlete. His training included mostly endurance conditioning, but he had never properly strengthened the back muscles or developed proper postural coordination. One day he bent over to lift a trash can, and "snap." A disc completely ruptured and the athlete ended up with a painful injury that required surgery. Before the injury, he had felt fine but his back was already in a weakened condition, with one or more of the discs taking the brunt of the load of many years of exercise and daily living.

At this point, the athlete was quite confused. "But, Doc, all I did was take out the trash. How could this have happened to me? After all, I'm in top condition!"

Although his legs and arms and cardiovascular respiratory systems had been developed and strengthened, this athlete had not been aware of the need to properly train and condition the back muscles to enable them to absorb the impact and load demanded by athletic participation. Being fit and healthy involves the body as a whole. It is not enough to properly develop part of the body if another is ignored. The back muscles are used each day by athletes and non-athletes alike. **To ignore the need to develop proper postural strength and coordination is to ignore a very important aspect of fitness.**

### CERVICAL SPINE

The *cervical* part of the spine, consisting of seven vertebrae, has a similar anatomy to the rest of the spine. It has vertebral bodies separated by intervertebral discs with nerve roots exiting through the *foramina* (round tunnels between each vertebra) on each side of the spine, at each level. At each of these levels, there are two *facet joints*—one on each side—and a *spinous process*.

*Cervical sprain* means there has been injury to the ligaments. It can be acute, caused by a blow, tearing the ligaments and resulting in swelling, pain and secondary muscle spasm. Or, it can be a chronic sprain where the ligaments have been stretched over a long period of time, resulting in secondary muscle spasm. Headaches as well as pain in the upper back can result from *chronic cervical strain*. This can be caused when the head (weighing about seven pounds) is not held in proper position by the neck muscles, requiring more tension to hold it up. Injuries to the spine are frequently termed "strain-sprain" because most of the time there are both ligament sprains and muscle strains, resulting in pain and muscle spasm.

Injuries to the disc in the cervical area frequently cause pain into the shoulder and arm and sometimes numbness into the upper extremity. In severe cases, weakness and numbness in the arms can result. Catastrophic injuries to the cervical spine such as a fracture which injures the spinal cord at that level can cause nerve damage and paralysis from the neck down. Injuries to the spinal cord high up in the cervical area usually cause death by cessation of breathing.

*Thoracic spine injuries* are similar both to the lumbar and cervical spine injuries in that they can also have a strain-sprain. Intervertebral disc ruptures in the thoracic spine are not as frequent because the thoracic spine is supported more by the chest and the ribs. Therefore, there is more stability to this area of the spine. This added support makes injuries to the thoracic spine less common.

Fractures of the neck and back are serious. Although they do not always result in paralysis, such an injury should always be treated as soon as possible by a medical specialist.

*Scoliosis* is the lateral curvature of the spine. It occurs in about five percent of children in the normal population. Though the origin of scoliosis is unknown, if detected, it should certainly be seen by a medical professional and evaluated for appropriate treatment. Without treatment, the curvature will usually progress.

Over 200 inner-city eight-to twelve-year-old children came together to spend part of their summer in an organized sports program. We developed the volunteer medical team to provide complete physical examinations and to treat any problems that might be found. It was estimated that 60% of these children had not been examined by a doctor since birth and many had somehow missed the various school health screenings. During these physicals, we diagnosed quite a few problems, including several cases of scoliosis. Although schools do scoliosis screening, it is still possible for children with scoliosis, as well as other serious problems, to slip through the system and go undetected. Sports programs requiring complete physical examinations can be very helpful in early detection of scoliosis and other possible problems.

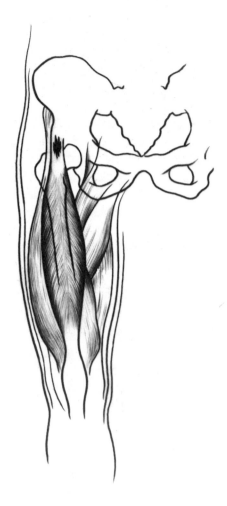

*This diagram illustrates a groin injury, in this case a tear of the rectus muscle at the hip, giving pain in the groin. Other areas of muscle attachment give pain in the groin. Bursitis can also give pain in the hip area.*

## INJURIES TO THE HIP AND GROIN

The hip muscles must be strong and coordinated, since they are important in maintaining body balance. Injuries to the hip and groin are frequently complex problems. An injury occurring in the hip area may be difficult to treat with rest because the muscles in the hip and groin never rest when the body is in a standing position. One of the largest muscles that flexes the hip, the *ilio-psoas*, originates in the low back, runs along the spine, through the pelvis, and attaches in the approximal femur. This muscle is important in maintaining posture in the lower back. Therefore, injuries in the lower back can cause pain and weakness in the hip.

Sometimes hip and groin complaints are hard to pinpoint. Because the hip and pelvis are close to the internal organs, pain in the hip can come from problems that are not musculoskeletal in origin, such as a hernia, entrapment of nerves, infection, and tumors.

Then, too, pain in the hip can be caused by serious problems in the skeleton, such as arthritis or stress fractures of the hip. Stress fractures in the hip can become severe problems. If the stress fractures are allowed to develop into complete fractures, the blood supply into the hip can be lost. This will cause a complete breakdown of the hip and require surgery, possibly even replacement of the hip. The prognosis in such a case is not good.

More frequent and less serious problems that cause hip pain are inflammation of either the *adductor longus muscle*, *rectus femoris muscle* or *ilio-psoas muscle*. Tears of these muscles are a more serious problem, especially the tear or rupture of the adductor longus muscle, since the adductor can rupture and tear off a piece of bone. Inflammation of these areas can frequently be treated with localized ice and anti-inflammatory medications. Most important, is working on the coordination and flexibility to the hip while the healing takes place, eliminating the original cause of the injury.

Ruptures or tears of the muscle attachments can usually be treated with rest, but surgery is sometimes necessary in complete ruptures. Persistent pain in the hip and joint area should always be checked by a professional to rule out more serious problems.

Other conditions that can cause pain that is felt in the hip or pelvis area are: appendicitis, *prosicitis* (infection or inflammation of the prostate gland), urinary tract infection, tumors, sciatica and bursitis. Difficulties with the pubic bone can be felt in the groin. For example, *osteitis pubis*, a stress injury where the two pubic bones meet to form the pelvic ring in the anterior part of the pelvis, may be felt as pain located in the front of the pubic bone. This sometimes shows up in x-rays.

*Trochanteric bursitis*, or inflammation over the trochanter is bursitis in the hip area, a frequent cause of pain especially on the lateral aspect (outside of the hip). Pain in the posterior aspect of the hip is sometimes caused by sciatica.

Like James Bond, you need to always be on the alert. No, not for bad guys, but for warning signs. The key to keeping your spine and the rest of your body healthy is to always be on a constant alert. A sudden, low backache? A sharp, throbbing pain down your side? Something that feels a heckuva lot like sciatica? Don't fool around! See a specialist and 007 that pain right now!

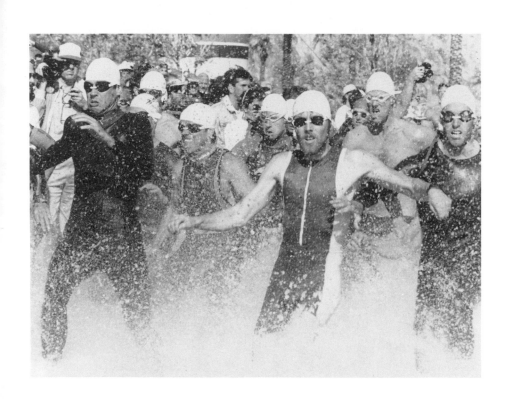

# Protection From the Elements

## Chapter Eleven
# Protection From the Elements

You live in Michigan and you've trained for a particular marathon all winter long. Early morning runs through the snow. Evening weight workouts at the club. You've trained for hills, for distance, and for speed. If someone looked up *prepared* in the dictionary, your smiling picture would be right there staring back at them. Race day finally comes and wouldn't you know it. It is <u>very</u> hot and <u>very</u> humid and five miles into the Los Angeles Marathon, it becomes obvious to you that the only way you're going to see the finish line is either from the medical tent or from the back seat of a taxi.

How did you mess up, Bunky? Here's a hint: It begins with a W, ends with an R and the letters "e" "a" and "t" play prominent roles. Give up? Well, the word is *weather*, and if you don't take it into account when you train or race you can bet that it will eat you up ....and spit you out.

Many of you remember watching TV during the '84 Olympics, when Gabrielle Anderson came staggering across the finish line in the women's marathon. She was suffering from a heat disorder.

As warm-blooded creatures, we need to maintain a near-constant core body temperature. When the body exceeds its capacity to regulate its temperature, problems result. Variation of core body temperature for an extended period of time can cause brain damage or even death.

With exercise, the muscles contract and heat is produced. As the blood is circulated through the muscles the blood warms. The heat is dissipated by cooling through sweat evaporation through the lungs. The body's heat regulator mechanism works by channeling blood to the skin's subcutaneous blood vessels that dilate to give more bloodflow. The sweat evaporation cools both skin and blood. This can become a problem when there is high humidity because, although the temperature is high, sweat cannot evaporate on the skin. Moisture evaporation from the lungs also aids in cooling the body. Dehydration can occur if the water loss is not replaced during exercise.

When working at peak efficiency, the body is truly amazing in adapting to extreme environmental changes. This is most evident in the performance of a trained and healthy athlete. Scott Molina, 1988 winner of the Hawaiian Ironman Triathlon (2.4 mile swim, 112 mile bike, 26.2 mile run), was standing with a group of reporters within minutes of finishing the race. He had just been asked by one of the journalists about how he had been training to get ready for an event that took eight and a half hours to finish and forced him to deal with the tough Hawaiian tradewinds and the 100 degree heat and humidity that makes the Ironman so darn humbling.

He paused momentarily to gather his thoughts. "Well, I'd like to tell you about my training," he said with a smile, "but I'd also like to be known as a relatively intelligent human being." Since Molina had always been troubled in the past when he tried to race in the heat, he spent 10 days in Palm Springs prior to Hawaii, riding and running as much as 10 hours a day, adapting his body to the high temperatures of the desert and, consequently, to the high temperatures of Ironman.

Under normal circumstances, the body is able to regulate itself, and like Scott Molina, adapt to unusual environments and trauma. Given the proper education and conditioning, the body is truly amazing in its ability to adapt to environmental extremes, but there is a limit—and each of us has his own. Exceed it and problems result.

## HEAT INJURY SYNDROME

If exercise plus environmental factors cause the body temperature to rise higher than the regulatory mechanisms can handle, heat injuries occur. One type of heat injury is heat cramps. The exact mechanism causing heat cramps is not well understood, but it seems to be associated with inadequate hydration.

## HEAT FATIGUE

Heat fatigue is seen in athletes who are not acclimatized to exercise in warmer environments or in environments with higher humidity. This is usually characterized by an earlier onset of fatigue and slower recovery from exercise. This is not serious, but should be a warning to decrease the intensity and length of exercise. Remember to hydrate with adequate replacement fluids.

## HEAT EXHAUSTION

The symptoms of heat exhaustion are dizziness, light-headedness, fatigue and weakness. The athlete may collapse due to a sudden drop in blood pressure. The rectal temperature is below 41 degrees centigrade or 105 degrees Fahrenheit. The skin is cool and sweating profusely. The athlete should be treated with replacement fluids, rest, and sometimes I.V. fluids.

## HEAT STROKE

Heat stroke is serious and truly a medical emergency. Rising body temperature and dry skin are characteristic signs. The patient may be incoherent and disoriented. If the rectal temperature taken is above 105.8 degrees Fahrenheit, the patient is assumed to have heat stroke. Treatment, including cooling with wet ice towels and I.V. fluid replacement, should be immediate. The patient should be removed to an emergency room as quickly as possible. The name of the game in treating this injury is to cool the body as rapidly as possible and replace fluids.

## COLD INJURIES

Cold injuries can come in two forms: *peripheral cold injuries* or frostbite and *central cold injuries* such as generalized hypothermia. One important thing to remember is that vigorous exercising in the cold can elevate body temperature as much as twenty-fold. Therefore, it is important to continue vigorous exercise as long as possible until appropriate shelter is found. Cold injuries are commonly seen when extreme cold is accompanied by high winds.

Education is important in preventing cold injuries. It is essential to insulate the extremities with gloves, and cover the head. A good rule of thumb: if you are cold, cover your head.

The head is more susceptible if it's wet and cold, as this is where about 30% of the body's heat is lost. The nose, ears, cheeks, fingers and toes, which are susceptible to frostbite, should be covered. Areas showing early signs of frostbite should be slowly warmed. Do <u>NOT</u> massage these extremities. The patient should be placed in a warm bath at 40 to 42 degrees centigrade and be seen by a professional.

*Hypothermia* is when the body temperature is lower than it should be due to exposure to the cold. Cold-related problems are some of the most common environmental injuries and can be the most severe, since the end result of severe hypothermia can be death. You don't have to be caught without clothes in a blizzard to have this happen. Healthy athletes have died from severe hypothermia resulting from cold water swims in triathlons. Remember that water conducts heat better than air. Therefore you lose heat much faster when you are wet. People who have very little body fat lose heat faster than those who have a layer of fatty insulation. Shivering is an automatic response of the body to preserve heat. Shivering is an indication of hypothermia.

# Wind Chill Factor Chart

| Wind Speed (mph) | Local Temperature (°F) Equivalent Temperature (°F) | | | | | | | | | | |
|---|---|---|---|---|---|---|---|---|---|---|---|
| | 32 | 23 | 14 | 5 | -4 | -13 | -22 | -31 | -40 | -49 | -58 |
| Calm | 32 | 23 | 14 | 5 | -4 | -13 | -22 | -31 | -40 | -49 | -58 |
| 5 | 29 | 20 | 10 | 1 | -9 | -18 | -28 | -37 | -47 | -56 | -65 |
| 10 | 18 | 7 | -4 | -15 | -26 | -37 | -48 | -59 | -70 | -81 | -92 |
| 15 | 13 | -1 | -13 | -25 | -37 | -49 | -61 | -73 | -85 | -97 | -109 |
| 20 | 7 | -6 | -19 | -32 | -44 | -57 | -70 | -83 | -96 | -109 | -121 |
| 25 | 3 | -10 | -24 | -37 | -50 | -64 | -77 | -90 | -104 | -117 | -130 |
| 30 | 1 | -13 | -27 | -41 | -54 | -68 | -82 | -97 | -109 | -123 | -137 |
| 35 | -1 | -15 | -29 | -43 | -57 | -71 | -85 | -99 | -113 | -127 | -142 |
| 40 | -3 | -17 | -31 | -45 | -59 | -74 | -87 | -102 | -116 | -131 | -145 |
| 45 | -3 | -18 | -32 | -46 | -61 | -75 | -89 | -104 | -118 | -132 | -147 |
| 50 | -4 | -18 | -33 | -47 | -62 | -76 | -91 | -105 | -120 | -134 | -148 |

*Little danger for properly clothed persons** — *Considerable danger** — *Very great danger**

*Danger from freezing of exposed flesh
Source: Courtesy U.S. Army Antarctic Research Laboratory, Chart 20-12.

Body functions, especially nerve and muscle function are greatly affected by cold temperatures. Shivering inhibits performance and also uses energy. The colder the environment, the more oxygen consumption is necessary to continue exercise. Therefore, fatigue occurs earlier and efficiency is decreased. It is obvious why this is true, since some of the body's energy is required to maintain heat. If the body temperature falls below 95 degrees Fahrenheit, mental functioning is impaired. Confusion is an indication of severe hypothermia.

Obviously, the best protection against hypothermia is appropriate clothing. Wearing clothing in layers is a better insulator. Also the fabric should be something that allows the skin to breathe, evaporating the sweat, thereby keeping the skin dry. Previously, one of the best materials for this was silk used in long underwear and turtlenecks. More recently, the newer synthetic fabrics are especially designed for this purpose and actually are as good or better than silk.

Severe hypothermia should be treated in a hospital. This occurs when the patient's core temperature is below 35 degrees centigrade or 95 degrees Fahrenheit.

"I remember the day like it was yesterday. The race billed itself as a national championship and was held the week after the Ironman Triathlon at Zuma Beach in Malibu in October of 1982. The event was nationally televised live on CBS, and as I swam what was supposed to be 1.5 miles in 65-degree water, early on I could feel my arms getting numb and my thoughts starting to wander. We found out afterwards that the water was 57 degrees and the swim was actually closer to two miles. Over 130 triathletes started the race but nearly 40 had to be pulled from the ocean by the lifeguards. Luckily, I had made it to shore, but when I did I remember yelling 'Where are the bikes! Where are the bikes!' They were actually about 50 yards in front of me, but my vision was so foggy that I couldn't identify anything! The next thing I remember is being led towards a warming hut so that I could get my temperature up, stop shivering and regain use of my senses. As I was being led away, a CBS camera crew came up and stuck a microphone under my nose. Without thinking I said 'Excuse me, I can't talk right now...I have a reservation at the Hypothermia Hotel.' To my ears, I sounded just fine. But when I saw the outtakes of the program later on that week, I was shocked. I realized then that I sounded more like someone who had just polished off a fifth of Jack Daniels^R than someone who was just a tad chilly. 'Exxxxxcuuuuuseee-mmmeeeeee,' I stammered, 'III caaaaannn't taaa-lllk riiiight nnnnoww, III haaave aa rrrresssser-vaatioon aaatt tthhee Hyyyppoooothermiiia Ho-tttel' That's when I first realized just how scary hypothermia can be."

Bob Babbitt, *Competitor Magazine*

## PROTECT YOURSELF FROM THE SUN

With an increasing loss of our ozone layer, which protects us from ultraviolet rays, there is an increase in the amount of skin damage secondary to sun exposure. Repeated episodes of damage can result in skin cancer. It is no longer "IN" to be exposed to the sun without some form of sun protection. If you must, you can still get a tan while protecting your skin from significant damage. If you do not use skin protection (and you get lucky) you may not get skin cancer—but you certainly will cause damage that will prematurely age your skin, making it less attractive.

Skin protection should especially be considered at higher altitudes and whenever snow or water reflection are a factor. Sunburn can be first- second- and third-degree. In a first-degree burn, the skin is red. This is superficial and will heal in a few days. In a second-degree burn, blisters form on the skin. This should be treated by a physician. A third-degree burn destroys skin layers. The victim should receive immediate medical attention by a physician.

Too much sun can obviously be harmful and for some people, even a little can do damage. **Use sun block.** Protect your skin from exposure to the harmful ultraviolet rays. This means your face, nose and lips, arms and hands, legs, chest and back—and yes, even the patch of skin on top of your head where your hair used to be.

Do it before you go out and if you will be exposed for awhile, bring along a mini-tube if you can. Since you will probably be sweating while you work out, perspiration-proof or waterproof brands might help a little more.

Also remember that at higher altitudes, near the water, or in the snow, the sun's rays are more intense. Protect yourself even more—and more often as the day goes on.

Wear a hat or a visor and good quality sunglasses. Protect your eyes from the sun and its reflection off the snow or water. If there is no snow or water around—protect them anyway. They are sensitive and can be damaged.

Now that you are working hard to keep your body in condition and fit, allow yourself the little extra time to protect your skin and keep it young and healthy and protect your eyes so you'll be able to see the good work you've done.

## INJURIES ASSOCIATED WITH HIGH ALTITUDES

Since there is less available oxygen at high altitudes, the athlete who is not acclimatized to higher altitudes will not be able to transport as much oxygen to the tissues. Therefore, your ability to perform aerobic workouts is decreased. You will then fatigue sooner due to lactic acid build-up. After two to four weeks at high altitude, your *hemoglobin* (number of red cells) will increase, increasing the amount of oxygen transported to the tissues. As that happens, the amount of exercise can be increased before fatigue sets in.

Altitude sickness is commonly observed in persons living in lower altitudes who go to higher altitudes such as ski areas. When the elevation level reaches about 5000 feet, *hypoxia* (lack of oxygen) is noticed significantly, especially with exercise. The first symptom of hypoxia would be hyperventilation or breathlessness. You may notice that mental tasks are more difficult, since mental alertness may be significantly decreased. Vision can be effected due to the lack of oxygen, and sleeping is sometimes disturbed.

The effects of alcohol, on the non-acclimated person are increased. It is not uncommon for people from a city at sea level to arrive at a ski area 8,000 feet above sea level, down a couple of drinks, zoom up to the top most run, bend over to adjust their straps only to pass out as they straighten themselves up. As you might have guessed, that, too, is one of the ways that high altitude can "get you."

## AIR POLLUTION

Pollutants in the air we breathe include oxides, ozone and carbon monoxide, oxides of nitrogen and oxides of sulfur. If you exercise outside in the city, it is wise to watch the pollution standard index published by the Environmental Protection Agency. If any of the pollutants exceed 200, you might give serious thought to skipping your outside exercise and move indoors for your workout.

Whether you train recreationally or seriously, you'll always want to remember our Sports Medicine motto: Be Prepared! Sound familiar? Well, it should. Like any good scout, be prepared for any weather condition that may arise. And like someone who plans on working out for the next 25 or 30 years or more, protect yourself from the elements by using sunscreen, sunglasses, a wetsuit where appropriate...and good old common sense.

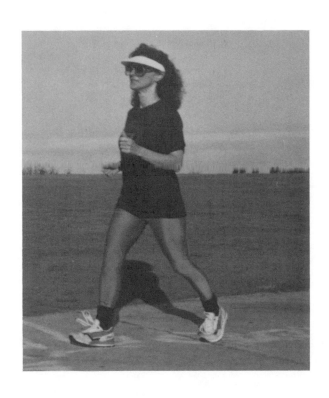

# The Beginning Athlete

# The Beginning Athlete

**To Begin** (*be-gin'*) *v.* 1. To commence, to initiate, to start. 2. To get off one's butt and work out.

The benefits derived from exercise are more than mere statistics can detail. People who keep fit are healthier, feel better, are happier and live longer. Governments and businesses have begun to realize that morale is higher and their employees tend to work better when they are fit, and their production goes up as a result.

In Japan, one of the leading nations in world production, busy companies include exercise periods as part of each work day. Some spend as much as 45 minutes a day to keep their employees fit.

We could be a much fitter and more productive nation if we adopted national and corporate pride in exercising and staying in shape. It is not that we haven't tried. Industrial fitness programs have been instituted from time to time, to get people in shape, promote corporate pride and increase productivity. Unfortunately, they are often abandoned because of the high injury rate that frequently results. Why does this happen? Mostly these programs do not address themselves to that very unique athlete—perhaps the most vulnerable of them all—The Beginning Athlete. The beginning athlete is usually not knowledgeable as to how the body works, the types of injuries that can occur or what to do to prevent these injuries. **And, in many cases, the beginning athlete ends up doing too much, too soon.**

The goal in exercise programs should not be to have "everyone involved running three miles by the end of the month." The real goal in any exercise program should be to avoid injury and promote well-being and better health.

The formula for a happy, pain-free beginning athlete is not difficult:

1. Start slowly.
2. Be gentle with your body.
3. Work out regularly and
4. Increase your activity at a slow and even pace.

Before a baby begins to run, it must first learn to walk. Before walking, that same baby spends months just kicking, rolling around, stretching, and maintaining flexibility before standing and taking that first step.

**Start slowly.** Remember that your body needs time to adjust to the new demands being made. Just because your brain says, "I want to be a runner," does not mean that your body is conditioned to do this without injury.

**Be gentle with your body.** Always warm-up before exercising. Stretch gently and "wake-up" and "warm-up" your muscles before starting. "Cool-down" and gently stretch when you finish. This takes very little time and can help keep you free from injury.

**Work out regularly.** Set a schedule and keep to it. Allow your body to get "used to" the regular routine of working out. Not only will you begin to look forward to your workout, you will be in a better position to **increase your activity at a slow and even pace.** The slower you increase your activity, the better your body's ability to meet the new demands without becoming injured. Finally, set a realistic time goal. If you are a beginning athlete, know that it should take at least one full month of a consistent 30-40 minute walking program before you begin to run. Take it slow and allow your body the time and conditioning it needs to proceed on your program, happily and without injury.

**The journey of a thousand miles
begins with a single step**

**Lao-tse**

## THE BEGINNING ATHLETE'S PROGRAM

1. **Follow the Warm-up Set of Exercises, noting any variations you may need to follow. Do them slowly, following the guidelines.**
2. **Follow the Beginner's Cardiovascular Exercise Plan.**
3. **Cool-down with the Stretching/Strengthening Set of Exercises, noting those variations you may need to follow.**

Helpful Hints for the Cardiovascular Exercise Plan:
1. Be sure that your socks and shoes are of a better quality and that your shoes are designed for exercise walking or running. This will give you the maximum cushion between you and the pavement.

2. Protect your skin from the sun. Use sun block. Shade your eyes for protection as well as comfort.

3. **WARM-UP!** Do The Warm-up Set of exercises noting any variations that may pertain to you. (*See Chapter Four, Individual Training Program.*)

4. Practice good posture while you walk. Remember, the muscles you use are the muscles you are strengthening. If you slouch or hunch, you could be setting yourself up for problems.

5. Walk at a smooth and consistent pace, increasing the pace as is comfortable. Remember, you are conditioning your body—not window shopping.

6. Time yourself. This way you can gradually lead up to a 30-40 minute walk, if you need to. Also, you will be able to time your "Run/Walk Schedule," should you choose to include it.

7. Gradually condition your body to walk any hills you may encounter. **Take it slow.** Some hills are formidable. Do a little at a time. Allow yourself one to two weeks, if needed. Avoid surprising your body with too much, too soon.

8. **Have fun!** This is your own, very private time. You are doing something just for **you!** So enjoy it.

9. When you are finished, cool-down with the Stretching/Strengthening Set of exercises and feel proud. **You have just become an Everyday Athlete.**

Since tendon and ligament tissues are most commonly the site of injuries, they should be given top priority. Emphasis should be put on exercising in such a way that the tendons and ligaments are protected and strengthened in order to reduce the risk of injury as much as possible. The Warm-up Set and a gradual progressive approach to your walking and/or running, will give you the best chance to accomplish this.

**I have met with but one or two persons in the course of my life who understood the art of walking. Every journey begins with the first step and every walk is a sort of crusade.**

—Henry David Thoreau

## THE BEGINNER'S CARDIOVASCULAR EXERCISE PLAN

If you haven't been on a *consistent* walking program in several months or more, it's important to start with a daily walk of 30-40 minutes and be consistent with that for at least a month before you consider starting a running program. You may even have to take time to build up to the 30-40 minute walk, depending on your condition. Remember, TAKE IT SLOW—you needn't be in a hurry to increase your program. After all, **with your first step on your first walk, you became an Everyday Athlete!** You may choose to follow the Beginning Athlete's Program with walking as your goal. This program, if done consistently, is fulfilling and rewarding and can give you a lifetime of fitness and well-being.

## BEGINNER'S 13-STEP PROGRESSIVE RUNNING PROGRAM

After following the walking program consistently for one month, you may choose to include running in your program. If you do, follow the Beginner's 13-Step Progressive Running Program, using the Run/Walk Schedule.

Always walk 8 to 10 minutes before you start your running sets, as part of your warm-up, and 10 minutes after your last run, as a cool-down. Walk for 2 minutes in between your running segments.

### Beginner's example:

Walk 10 minutes, run 1 minute, walk 2 minutes, run 1 minute, walk 2 minutes, run 1 minute, walk 10 minutes. Total 27 minutes.

# RUN/WALK SCHEDULE

## WALK/RUN
## (TIME IN MINUTES)

| | **WARM-UP** | | | | | **COOL-DOWN** | |
|---|---|---|---|---|---|---|---|
| **Level** | **Walk** | **Run** | **Walk** | **Run** | **Walk** | **Run** | **Walk** |
| 1 | 10 | 1 | 2 | 1 | 2 | 1 | 10-15 |
| 2 | 10 | 1 | 2 | 1 | 2 | 2 | 10-15 |
| 3 | 10 | 1 | 2 | 2 | 2 | 2 | 10-15 |
| 4 | 8-10 | 2 | 2 | 2 | 2 | 2 | 10 |
| 5 | 8-10 | 2 | 2 | 2 | 2 | 4 | 10 |
| 6 | 8-10 | 2 | 2 | 2 | 2 | 6 | 10 |
| 7 | 8-10 | 2 | 2 | 2 | 2 | 8 | 10 |
| 8 | 8-10 | 2 | 2 | 2 | 2 | 10 | 10 |
| 9 | 8-10 | 2 | 2 | 2 | 2 | 12 | 10 |
| 10 | 8-10 | 2 | 2 | 2 | 2 | 14 | 10 |
| 11 | 8-10 | 2 | 2 | 2 | 2 | 16 | 10 |
| 12 | 8-10 | 2 | 2 | 2 | 2 | 18 | 10 |
| 13 | 8-10 | | | | | 20 | 10 |

**BE SURE TO START AT THE BEGINNING.** Stay at each level for at least a week and Don't Skip Levels! It will take you at least 13 weeks to build up to a 20-minute run. If you have been a runner but you haven't been on a consistent running program for the last several months, it's important that you start slow and at a comfortable level and gradually build up the intensity (pace) and duration (number of minutes) of your runs. This may mean that you start at the beginning.

This may seem too cautious to you because your cardiovascular system will not be heavily challenged. But the emphasis in this approach is to build tendon and ligament strength as a priority, avoiding the most common injuries that runners are prone to, and you will be giving the Warm-up Set and Stretching/Strengthening Set a chance to strengthen the involved tissues as well.

After you lay a foundation with this conditioning program and build up your running time to 20 minutes and have done so consistently for one to two weeks, then you can gradually add five minutes every two weeks to your running time until you reach the number of minutes you want. Generally speaking, 20-30 minutes of running, three to four times a week is a good minimum to maintain good cardiovascular, respiratory health. But build up to that level slowly for the best results. Don't exceed the parameters of the heavy-light exercise schedule described in *Training and Conditioning*, and work out a maximum of six days per week.

Your body is an amazing thing and if conditioned properly and exercised regularly, will give you years of loyal service. It is your responsibility to treat it with care. Be gradual and gentle when asking it to do anything new. If you should feel pain at any time—remember your body is talking to you, telling you that something may be wrong. If the pain continues, listen carefully and seek help from your Sports Medicine Team. The key to continuing success for the Everyday Athlete is to be honest with yourself and be proud to start at the Beginning.

**To Continue** *(kon-tin'yoo) v.* 1. To last, to go on with, to endure. 2. To walk when you don't feel like it, to swim when the water looks too cold, to run when you'd rather not...**to stay fit for life!**

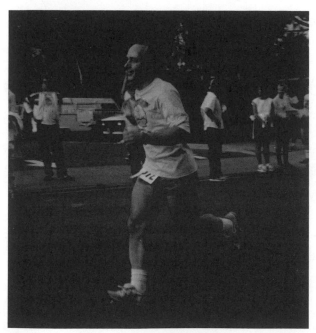

*Starting over after a serious knee injury, I used the guidelines perivouly illustrated. After four and a half months, I ran my first 10 K -- painfree.*

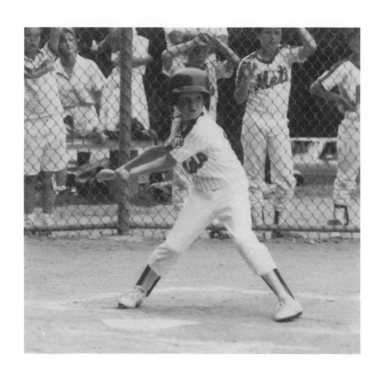

**Chapter Thirteen**
# Exercise and the Young Athlete

## Chapter Thirteen
# Exercise and The Young Athlete

It was the final game of the Little League season, the crowd was hushed and the bases were loaded. With two strikes already against him, the batter was under considerable pressure. The coach was visibly perspiring and both teams were as tense as they could be when all of a sudden, a woman's voice from the bleachers shouted, "It's OK, baby, just do the best you can."

With this message of encouragement, the silence had been broken. The crowd visibly relaxed, both the pitcher and the batter smiled, the pitch was made and the game, once again, became the FUN it was always intended to be.

"Just do the best you can." Now that's something you wouldn't hear a Major League player's mom yell at a National League pennant game. But kids are different, even when they are competing in the same sports as Mom and Dad. While every athlete needs support, a young athlete needs more—more support, more love and more understanding.

## EXERCISE AND THE YOUNG ATHLETE

It is important to understand that children are not just small adults or scaled-down versions of the full-size model. There are certain things about growth and development which should be taken into consideration when evaluating an exercise or sports activity for young people who have not yet reached their full growth potential.

When bones, tendons, ligaments and cartilage are growing, injuries can occur which can effect young people, causing a permanent deformity such as injury to the growth plate.

On the other hand, it has been shown that fitness in childhood, both musculoskeletal and cardiovascular, leads to a healthier, more satisfactory adult life. With a well-designed exercise program, injuries can be prevented. It is important for parents, coaches, trainers, teachers and the young athletes as well, to understand the basics of a good fitness program.

## SKELETAL GROWTH

From the time we are born until the time we reach full skeletal maturity (in the teenage years), the bones of the body are growing. During this time, they are composed of living cells, which are constantly dividing and multiplying and reshaping the bone. These small cells are surrounded by a material called the *matrix*. This matrix is incorporated with calcium to give the bone its hardness. The long bones of the body, those bones that form the extremities (the arms and legs), grow in length and width until skeletal maturity is reached.

In these bones, growth occurs from a remarkable structure called a *growth plate*. As long as the growth plate is active, bone growth will continue. An active growth plate marks the difference between childhood and adulthood, as far as skeletal injuries are concerned.

The growth plate is not easily injured in the normal running and jumping stresses of childhood. However, excessive stresses across the growth plate, or breaks in the growth plate, can cause it to stop growing altogether or to grow in an abnormal manner, causing a deformity. Surrounding the growing bone is cartilage, also immature and vulnerable to excessive stresses which can cause cartilage damage and deformity.

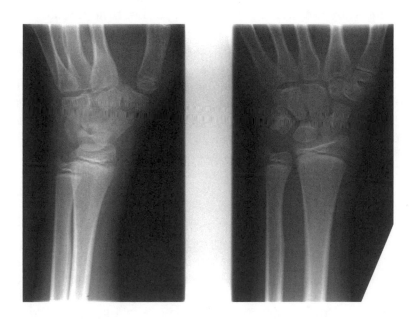

*This x-ray of the long bone of a child shows the growth plate with the epiphysis and the metaphysis.*

Initially, our skeletal framework consists entirely of cartilage. This is converted to bone by a process called *ossification* (making of bone). After primary ossification, skeletal growth continues by continuously breaking down, reshaping and adding new bone. Some ossification takes place by first going through a cartilage growth phase and then converting the cartilage to bone. This takes place at the physis and epiphysis and is responsible for the growth in the <u>length</u> of long bones (arms and legs).

There is another form of ossification responsible for the growth in <u>width</u> of long bones and also the growth of flat bones (pelvis and skull). In this form, bone is created directly, without a cartilage phase.

There are many differences between bone and cartilage tissue. Bone tissue is harder and stronger and contains calcium. X-rays show the bone because of the calcium content.

The growth plate is the clear area seen between the two calcified, bony areas. No calcium has yet been deposited on the growth plate, so it appears clear on the x-ray.

The word *"epiphysis"* comes from the Greek words *physis,* which means *growth*, and *epi*, which means *upon*. The epiphysis is the cap-like portion above the growth plate. The *epiphysis* means "upon the growth plate." *Meta* in Greek means *after.* *Metaphysis* means "after the growth plate." *Apo* means *offshoot*, and *apophysis* is a growth plate that appears as an offshoot from the bone.

The apophysis growth area is where a muscle-tendon attaches to bone. Prior to full growth, this is frequently an area of injury. When the forces across a muscle-tendon unit are too strong, the apophysis can be pulled away from bone, as in Osgood-Schlatter's disease. Generally, active growth plates are more susceptible to injury than joint ligaments. Growth plates are usually weaker than the ligaments prior to the closure of the growth plates, so it is important to evaluate the growth areas of the bone when an injury near the joint is suspected. **Over half of the fractures occuring in the pre-teen years involve a growth plate.** Once the growth plates are closed, injury to a joint is more likely to be a ligament injury or a sprain.

Most of the growth plate injuries will heal without complications if protected and no further injury occurs. But it is important to evaluate these kinds of injuries to avoid secondary growth problems. When a joint injury is involved, it is important to have an orthopedic surgeon who is familiar with these types of injuries evaluate the child.

## OSGOOD-SCHLATTER'S DISEASE

Many people have heard of Osgood-Schlatter's disease, a condition involving the growing attachment of the patellar tendon to the tibia (an *apophysis)*. The exact causes are unclear.

It seems to be a traction-stress type of injury, occurring in adolescence, in which a growing bone is pulled loose, causing inflammation. This will heal but may require casting. It seldom requires surgery. Physical therapy is important to regain the muscle coordination and strength after the inflammation has settled down.

## LITTLE LEAGUE ELBOW

"Little League" elbow, unfortunately a common injury, effects 12-20% of young pitchers. It is a serious injury that can easily be prevented. (*See Chapter Nine, Upper Extremity.*)

## TRAINING AND CONDITIONING

Fitness in childhood is very profitable and positive. We know that physically fit children will, in general, do better in sports activities. When a child is involved in a proper fitness program first, there is a decrease in the injury rate. **The child will enjoy sports more and get hurt less.**

## POSTURE

**A good postural strengthening and coordination program in childhood is one of the most important areas to emphasize, since it can lead to a healthier and injury-resistant adult.** If you watch babies sitting on the floor, you can see how they automatically sit with perfect posture, holding themselves erect. Notice their perfect flexibility. As children grow, however, their postural coordination becomes less automatic, and being great imitators, they will usually begin to mimic the posture of their parents or their role models. In more cases than not, children will then begin to develop poor postural habits.

Growing bones will respond to stresses and extremes in poor posture. This can cause abnormal growth of bones due to the abnormal stresses.

Most of us know that merely telling a child, "Sit up straight," "Don't slouch," or "Pull your shoulders back" is not effective. What *is* effective is to have good role models who demonstrate perfect posture. Talk to your children about the importance of good posture. Discuss how this can help them not only look better but become better athletes who are less likely to get hurt. Make postural exercises a regular form of exercise. If the parents understand this, the children will too. If the parents do these postural exercises, the children will do them as well.

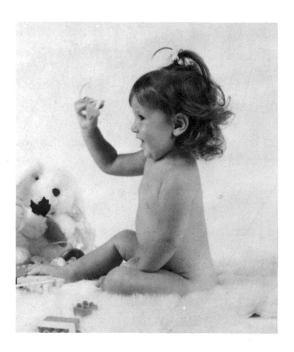

*Note the perfect posture that comes automatically in a young child. We are born with good posture. What happens?*

## FLEXIBILITY

Flexibility exercises for children are important. If flexibility training is maintained throughout childhood, the liklihood of injury is decreased. **Flexibility and postural strengthening exercises should be as much a part of everyday activity as brushing your teeth.**

## MUSCLE STRENGTH

Muscle strength in children will definitely improve with strength training. This can happen naturally with a regular exercise program and athletics. It's important to very carefully monitor any weight training prior to puberty. Weight training can be harmful due to joint overload on the ends of the long bones. If muscles are pulling too hard at the tendon bone attachment, they can pull off that vulnerable apophysis, causing abnormal growth in that area.

## OTHER PROBLEMS ASSOCIATED WITH GROWTH

Growth plates can be involved in problems other than direct injuries to the joint or stress injuries. There are diseases associated with the epiphysis in which it loses its blood supply. These problems require specialized treatment by an orthopedic surgeon. Any time a child is experiencing pain in a joint, he or she should be evaluated by a physician. Any time a child is limping, that child should be carefully observed. **If young athletes complain of pain, they should be listened to and evaluated.** Pain in a knee may actually be something going on with the hip. Any time swelling is seen around a joint, the child should be evaluated specifically.

## CHILDHOOD TRAINING AND CONDITIONING

### Pre-School Years
During these years, the exercises the child experiences should basically be things that are FUN—carefully created games to play and, hopefully, parents to share them with. Since children are great imitators, they will pick up traits by doing things with Mom and Dad. During these younger years, a regular endurance or strength program is not necessary. Instead, it is important to emphasize, through example and fun things to do, good posture, balance, coordination and flexibility.

### School Age
At this time, the child begins to enjoy more formal, more organized school experiences which should include organized and carefully monitored conditioning programs. Take care, though

—this should not be very competitive. Instead, make it something FUN, reinforcing the importance of a regular exercise program and a positive attitude toward exercise and fitness. Include agility training, push-ups and sit-ups. **Form is more important than strength.**

### Pre-Adolescent Years

During the years prior to puberty, training and conditioning programs can become more intense, more competitive, and last longer. It is important to remember, during this period of rapid growth, not to overstress the musculoskeletal system, causing growth plate injuries. Also, it is very important to emphasize flexibility and, again, a positive attitude.

### Teenage Years

As young athletes begin to mature, they develop greater strength and muscle mass. Weight training in this age group may have benefits, **but still should not be overdone.** It is important, going into this phase, that the child have good posture, flexibility and coordination. Remember, the muscles will respond to exercise, getting bigger and stronger. **The muscle patterns used in exercise and strength training will be strengthened.** Therefore, if teens are strengthening the wrong muscles, they can set themselves up for injuries down the road. In other words, **it's important to strengthen muscles while using good form.** This is true for athletes of any age. The body works more efficiently from the proper position. If you have good form going into a strengthening phase, you will not only have fewer injuries, but you will be a **better** athlete.

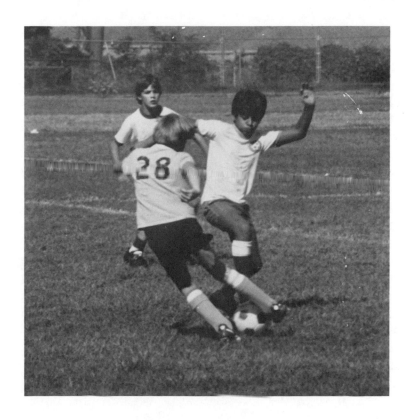

*Children in team sports.*

## SPORTS-SPECIFIC EXERCISES

In general, the earlier the child gains certain specific skills, the better he or she will perform in sports. At a very early age, children can begin sports activities that require coordination, timing, agility and balance. These activities should be fun and emphasize coordination rather than strength or endurance. For instance, children can begin skiing at pre-school age. These children can, with proper guidance, develop balance, agility, and coordination naturally. Still, these activities should be approached carefully to make sure the child does not develop an injury or become fearful. **Remember, pushing a child into an intensive program before the child is ready can be detrimental.**

Parents need to encourage children to do something with fitness every day. That way, they develop a pattern of regular exercise at an early age. It's important that physical activity be a regular part of their lives. It's important that they develop this attitude on their own, without a lot of pressure or stress, which could discourage them from exercising in the future. **Do not force a child to play when hurt.** Whether it is a physical or psychological problem is not important. **What is important is not to pressure children into playing when they don't feel like they should.**

When working with youngsters, try to remember back to our earlier example of the Little League players. The mom who yelled "It's OK baby, just do the best you can," was telling us something essential about children. Children's bodies—and psyches—while they might appear, on the outside, to be very adult-like in nature—are in reality very fragile...They need extra. Extra support, extra understanding and extra love to make it all work.

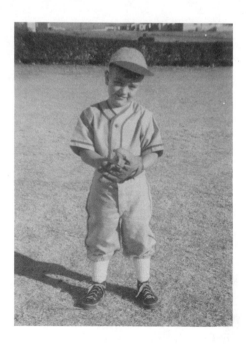

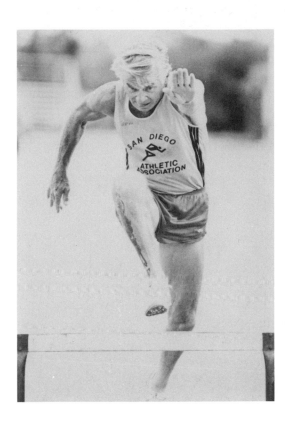

*Dr. Jock Jocoy...the 1984 National Pentathlon Champion and National Decathlon Champion. He set a world record in 1984 in Decathlon in his age category. He has been selected All-American several times, most recently in 1988-89 in the Decathlon.*

## Chapter Fourteen
# The Over Fifty Athlete

## Chapter Fourteen
# The Over Fifty Athlete

An over fifty, Everyday Athlete thinks back to childhood and remembers what "Old" meant then. Fifty-year-"old" women, back then wore thick, support hose, strange bulky shoes and were doubled over as they walked at a snail's pace. The men were bulging around the middle, puffing while climbing stairs and seemed to have a lot of trouble remembering things. You know, the ones seen slowly walking down to the corner store to get a pack of cigarettes or a cigar. "Ah, the good ole days," when fifty was **OLD** and anyone older was **ANCIENT**.

Well those days are long gone and to that we say "Good riddance!" Today, an over fifty athlete looks in the mirror and sees a younger, fitter body, the body of a healthy person, a body capable and eager for the coming years.

**So-what's-it-gonna-be-Buckaroos? Over fifty and active to the best of your body's ability or over fifty and <u>OLD</u>?**

What do you consider old? Seventy? Eighty? Maybe Ninety? It all depends on your point of view. There are whole groups of people, in several locations on earth, who live beyond a hundred years of age. Studies of the Ecuadoreans in Vacabamba or the Karakoram tribes in Kashmir or even the Russians in Abkagia, show that it is more than heredity that allows so many to live so long. They have healthy food habits—they take in no more than 1800 calories a day. They maintain good flexibility and conditioning by continuing to do arduous tasks, such as climbing mountains and moving rapidly through valleys on foot (doing so well past the age of eighty). Also, in their cultures it is the expectation that, with age, they continue to perform regular physical labor, keeping their bodies fit and their minds active. These are physically active people!

We can then compare the lifestyle of these people with that of the people of North America. We are a people who spend most of our time sitting...not walking, running or climbing. Our food habits include "junk foods," high fat intake, refined sugar and overeating. And we are still locked into the "retirement syndrome" of inactivity—a sure killer, or at least, a disabler of older people.

But this is an "old" trend and it is beginning to change. Instead, we are starting to watch what we eat and we are becoming aware of our bodies and what it takes to keep them healthy and fit.

We now have fine athletes greater than fifty years of age and more are joining the ranks every day. Some have moved all the way through their 70's and are still in great shape. **These are some of our most remarkable competitive as well as Everyday Athletes.**

One of my patients, a decathlon champion, has passed the 60-year mark. He didn't start participating in athletic events until he was in his fifties and had undergone surgery on his back. Of course, not everyone can win that kind of race, but anyone can be in better condition through a smart program of fitness.

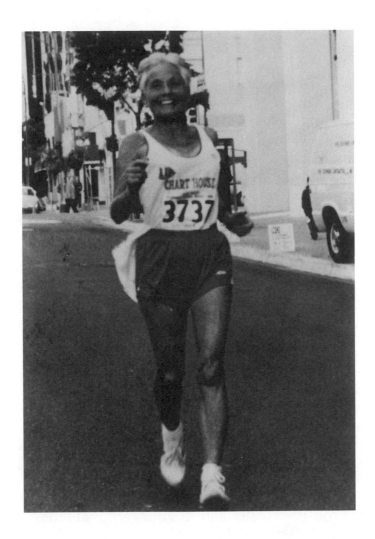

*Judy Simon started running while in her 50's. She was named Runner of the Year for age 70-74 for 1986, 87 by <u>Running Times</u> Magazine. She ran her first marathon at the age of 67. Now she is over 70 and younger every year. An exceptional athlete and a real winner!*

## THE OLDER ATHLETE

The older athlete moves better, thinks better, looks better and feels better than those who are "just-plain-older."

Over fifty athletes can have unusual strength, muscular endurance and good flexibility into, and beyond, the seventies bracket, if they follow a correct program of fitness instruction. Such a program may also assure better overall health than they would have had without regular exercise. When athletes continue to maintain a high level of fitness, the gradual decline in strength that usually comes with the added years (and has been so well documented by researchers) is postponed or avoided for a long period of time.

The secret is knowledge of the body and what it can endure. Of course there **MUST** be a medical exam before leaping into a fitness program. **Before starting an exercise program on a daily basis consult your doctor to determine the possible risks.** Even though there may be risks, it is still within the range of everyone to improve.

With the present trend toward more active middle-aged athletes, and as the middle-aged athlete becomes the older athlete, we find that there is a postponement of declining strength and endurance as individuals become better educated in training and conditioning, and in prevention of injuries.

From ages thirty to forty, the elasticity of tendons decreases or declines and bone strength decreases after age fifty. **We know that inactivity accelerates this degeneration.** Joints and the surrounding connective tissue age rapidly, and when not exercised on a regular basis, tendons, ligaments and joint capsules shorten and thicken and become difficult to stretch. Stiffness sets in and bending becomes a chore. **Disuse dramatically effects movement.**

Of course it is possible that a certain degree of wearing away of protective tissue and its lubricating abilities make it painful to do certain types of exercises. This is understandable, but it does not preclude a wide range of alternative exercises that can produce a fitness profile. Swimming is a good example. It relieves the body of weight-bearing stresses on bones and joints.

Many recent studies in medical literature have shown that middle-aged and older individuals who exercise regularly maintain higher levels of fitness and show superior levels of strength and endurance than those who do not. These athletes actually show higher levels of function and have a higher level of maximum oxygen uptake than younger individuals who do not exercise.

## FITNESS SPORTS FOR THE OVER FIFTY ATHLETE

There is a certain structural vulnerability in anyone who is older and participating in sports activities, and that vulnerability increases in one who is not conditioned. But there are activities that carry a lesser degree of potential injury. Many over fifty athletes participate in walking, running, swimming, tennis, cycling and other non-contact sports. These activities can be an exciting and beneficial way to retard the decline of strength, endurance and flexibility.

Perhaps one of the secrets to avoiding injuries is to avoid contact sports. Some elderly athletes need to avoid any sport that is combative or contact. For some, even tennis—which requires twisting and sudden movements—could cause injury. But for most who follow a carefully designed fitness program, even sports that require sudden starts and abrupt stops, twisting and rapid direction change, can be undertaken if proper stretching movements and exercises to condition the body for those movements have been part of the fitness program. **Careful assessment of capacities is essential to any participation in sports.** Also, for any athlete there is a readiness factor when beginning to participate in a sport. This needs to be assessed by your physician. A program to include certain exercises must be followed to ensure a degree of success and to avoid injuries. Again, take it slow. Follow the program designed just for you.

In anyone over sixty, there will be a certain amount of loss of flexibility, endurance and strength. This is part of nature and the decrements of the human body. Keep in mind, however, that regular exercise will minimize this process. Anyone over fifty who wishes to reach a "training effect" must do so with regular rhythmic exercises such as walking, running, cycling or swimming. For this to occur, the cardiovascular system must be in condition to deliver oxygen and nutrients to the working muscles, and the lungs must be able to provide adequate oxygen to the blood. Some sports require greater circulatory and respiratory efficiency than agility or muscle strength. All of these factors need to be considered in a specifically tailored program designed by your physician just for you.

So—What's it gonna be?

A. Baggy, thick support stockings, heavy clunky shoes, hunched back and a big pot belly? You know—barely able to walk up a flight of stairs without wheezing or gasping for air? In other words, **GROWING OLD!**

Or—Do you choose:

B. Staying active, looking good, staying fit and healthy—quick of mind with a conditioned, flexible body?

What's that you say—you choose **B**?

Congratulations! You've Won The Jackpot—and the prize: **A Quality of Life Worth its Weight in Gold!**

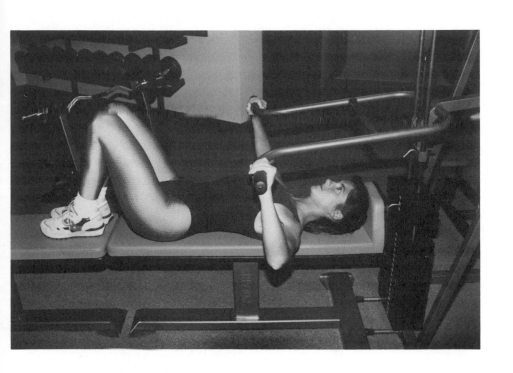

Chapter Fifteen
# The Indoor Athlete

## Chapter Fifteen
# The Indoor Athlete

The weather outside is frightful...but what the heck can you do indoors? Welcome to our new game, *Reader's Choice*:

If it's lousy outdoors, what would YOU do?

A) Move all the furniture?
B) Repaint the walls?
C) Wash the dishes?
D) Dust the blinds?
E) Clean out the attic?
F) Watch a MASH rerun and ride
   your stationary bicycle?

Now doesn't F sound like the best of the bunch? There's no law that says you have to get all your exercise outdoors. Welcome to the wonderful world of indoor training. Remember....being fit is **IN**.

Exercising indoors is not a new thing. It's been around as long as man has had sense enough to come in out of the rain, and has had a desire to exercise. What's new, of course, is the equipment available. Today, there is a large number of exercise and strengthening aids developed for indoor participation. And with the invention of the computer, exercise monitoring has taken on a whole new dimension, making it easier and less boring.

The important thing about choosing equipment to use at home is to make absolutely sure, before you buy, that it is something you will really use. Too many times a rowing machine or exercise bicycle ends up hanging in the garage. Either the type of exercise the machine provides is not interesting or fun, or the equipment is of inferior quality and is soon replaced by a better model.

Start at stores that specialize in exercise equipment. They can provide a wider selection in different price ranges, and they usually have trained professionals to help you select the equipment. Many times they will even help you develop an exercise program.

Be knowledgeable. Decide what will work for you, keeping certain questions in mind. What level of aerobic fitness would you like to accomplish? Do you plan to use this on a daily basis or is this equipment meant to be used seasonally? What specific area of the body do you want to exercise?

## AEROBIC TRAINING EQUIPMENT

The most common aerobic training aids are exercise bikes, rowing machines and treadmills. And don't forget the good old jump rope—a popular (and one of the cheapest) forms of indoor exercise equipment. Other popular forms of indoor aerobic exercise aids include stair-climbing machines, cross country ski machines, turbo trainers and multi-station gyms.

## EXERCISE BIKES

**Pros:** Exercise bikes can give excellent aerobic fitness and also strengthen the leg muscles. A fancy name for an exercise bike is *ergometer*. It is simply an exercise bike with some sort of monitoring device measuring the amount of work performed.

This is a good piece of equipment, as it provides a supplement to any exercise program. It is easy to use, less jarring to the body, relatively inexpensive and doesn't take up much space.

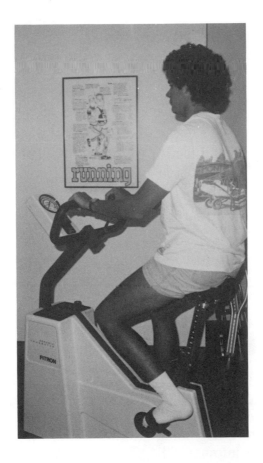

*Stationed in front of T.V. for decreasing boredom factor. Some more expensive models have complex computer programs to vary resistance. Several program selections are available.*

**Cons:** Like any indoor exercise machine, there is a boredom factor. This can be helped by watching television or reading a book while riding your "bike."

There are injuries associated with bike riding, including tendinitis in the knee, nerve compressions from pressure on the seat, back problems and nerve entrapments in the hand due to pressure on the hands. Back problems are more common with cyclists. The ergometer design which positions the body in an upright position, rather than bent over, causes fewer injuries of nerve entrapments of the hands and less back problems than traditional racing-style bicycles, while nerve compression due to the seat can be diminished by making sure that the seat is wide, well padded and fits the person using it.

**Helpful Hints:** When selecting your ergometer, be sure that it fits properly to your body. Anyone with a back problem should choose one with a back support or a reclined position. Look for a very heavy flywheel, which means a much more stable, quiet ride. It is also important to have sturdy, heavy-duty pedals with toe clips. Book racks are certainly not necessary, nor do they effect the quality of the equipment, but they may make your "ride" a little more fun.

**Training Tips:** For minimal aerobic training, cycling should be done three times a week for at least 30 minutes. The ideal speed is about 90 RPMs at a resistance that keeps your heart rate in the target zone that we have mentioned. To decrease boredom and improve your workout, vary the speed by increasing the RPMs or turning up the resistance. This will raise your pulse above the anaerobic threshold and increase your aerobic capacity while you build more muscle strength.

Adjust the equipment to suit your body. Adjust your seat so that in the downstroke your knee is not quite all the way extended. Adjust the handlebars so that when you lean forward you can keep your back straight.

If you are a beginning athlete and are just starting out on this type of equipment, TAKE IT SLOW. Start with a 10-15 minute exercise period at a moderate or low tension three times a week. Then add five minutes every two to three riding days so you can comfortably build up to the recommended times with a little heavier tension.

**Author's Recommendation:** Most ergometers are simple in design, while some come with computerized programs and even their own viewing screens. Although such extras can be helpful and fun, they are certainly not necessary. Just make sure the machine you buy is heavy-duty, stable, has a heavy flywheel, and that it at least measures RPMs and has an adequate timer. Such a machine should suit your purposes and provide many hours of indoor exercise. Wind resistance machines have certain advantages and should be considered.

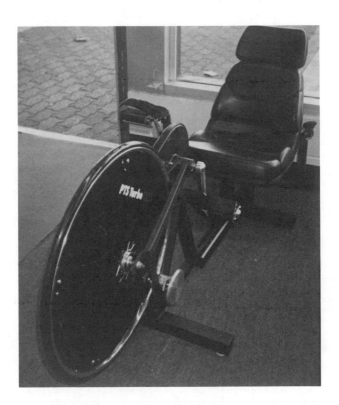

*Some models use wind resistance and provide back support.*

## TURBO TRAINERS

If you already have your own bicycle and wish to work out on it, but want the option of an indoor workout, buying an attachment called a Turbo Trainer is for you.

**Advantages**: These are relatively inexpensive and more sports-specific for cyclists, allowing them to get used to their own bicycle (especially the seat) while riding indoors.

**Helpful Hints:** Various attachments can be added to the Turbo Trainer. Videos are also available featuring The Tour de France[R] and the Coors Classic[R] so that the indoor riders can actually feel they are riding those race courses. And, if they like, they can even race a buddy!

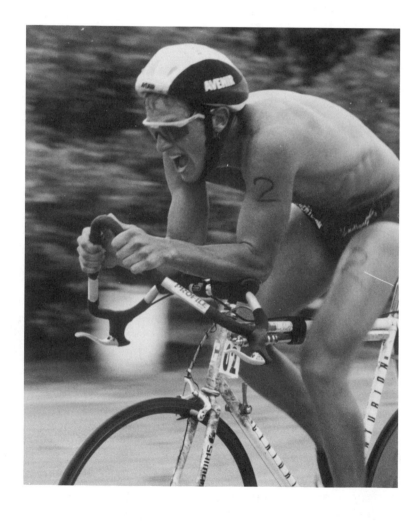

*Many competitive cyclists and triathletes train with turbo trainers, using their own custom fitted bikes.*

## TREADMILLS

**Pros:** Treadmills are excellent for training, especially for the person who likes to run but is not always able to run outside. They also have the advantage of decreasing the shock to your legs and back. You can keep an even pace on a treadmill and easily fall into a comfortable rhythm for your walk or run.

**Cons:** Treadmills take getting used to, even for the seasoned runner. Another disadvantage is that there is a tendency not to vary speed or stride length, which you normally do if you're running or walking outside. By slowing down or speeding up the machine, you can better simulate outdoor exercise.

**Helpful Hints**: If you plan to buy a treadmill, get a motorized one with a substantial motor (usually two and a half horsepower). In other words, one that's going to last!

## ROWING MACHINES

**Pros:** Rowing machines provide excellent workouts to both upper and lower extremities. Good for both anaerobic and aerobic training, they are durable and relatively inexpensive. These can also give strength training, endurance and aerobic and anaerobic fitness.

**Cons:** There is a higher incidence of back injury on rowing machines when inexperienced and beginning athletes use them before proper flexibility and coordination are achieved. Another cause for injury on a rowing machine is the lack of proper techniques. Some people buy the machine at a local store without receiving any explanation of its use. Also, boredom can be a problem with rowing machines just like with any other indoor exercise equipment.

**Helpful Hints:** Have a trained professional go through the proper technique with you before you buy. Also look for a heavy-duty model with a wide seat that is comfortable and has good stability.

**Training Suggestions**: When beginning on a rowing machine, it is important to start slowly—<u>much slower than starting on an exercise bike</u>. Begin with a moderate resistance workout, a two-minute workout with a two-minute break, going back for a total of six minutes. You can increase this two to four minutes each week until you reach a 30 minute workout, three times a week.

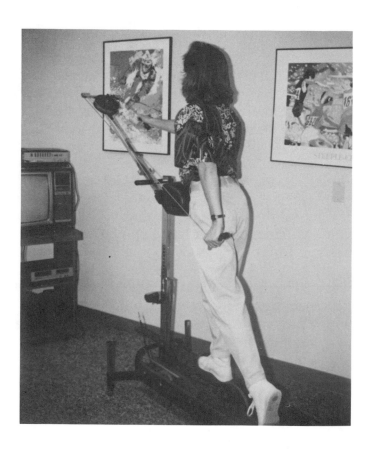

*Cross Country Ski Simulator*

## CROSS COUNTRY SKI SIMULATORS

**Pros:** Cross country skiing is one of the best methods for aerobic exercise. The cross country ski machine simulates the cross country ski motion and exercises both the upper body and the lower body without giving your legs and back the pounding they receive when running on pavement.

**Cons:** I have seen incidence of groin injuries associated with some of these machines. Also, a beginner may have difficulty, at first, developing the proper coordination and balance to exercise safely.

**Helpful Hints:** If you are going to buy a cross country ski machine, get a heavy-duty model. This could cost close to $500. Anything much lower in price may not withstand repetitive workouts. Some models are easier to use than others. Try them out before you invest in one.

## STAIR-CLIMBING MACHINES

**Pros:** Stair-climbing machines are a good form of aerobic exercise which strengthen the quadriceps and the buttocks muscles.

**Cons:** Anybody who has problems with inflammation of the knee should choose another form of exercise. Otherwise, it's a good source of strengthening and aerobic conditioning.

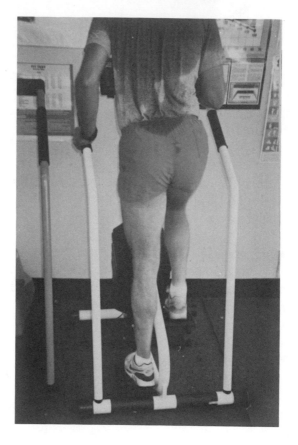

*Stair-climbing machine can be good aerobic exercise.*

## FREE WEIGHTS

**Pros:** The most common form of exercise aimed at building strength is free weights. Free weights are inexpensive and indestructible. Almost any muscle group can be exercised, and endurance training can also be accomplished. Some minimal aerobic workout can be attained, but generally free weights are used for strengthening, endurance, toning and body building.

**Cons:** Free weights cause more injuries than exercise machines. When doing heavy weights, it is important to have a friend nearby in case you need assistance. You should support your lower back at all times. When starting out, professional guidance is strongly recommended.

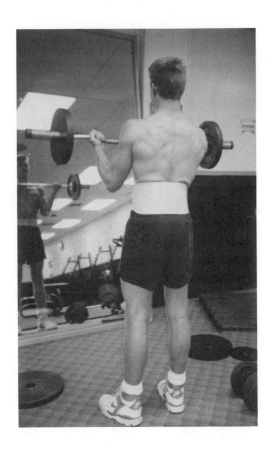

*Free Weights with back support*

**Training Suggestions:** After warming up, work first with the larger muscles and work down to the smaller muscles. Do your workouts every other day. If you lift every day, alternate the muscle groups you are exercising and give each a day of rest between workouts. If you are a beginner, start using a comfortable amount of resistance and gradually add weight. Strength building should be done by using three sets of four to ten repetitions at your maximum strength. For endurance, work at about 60% of your maximum strength for three sets, building up to 20 to 30 repetitions. Also, do sports-specific exercises (exercising the muscles you use in your sport) at a higher speed, trying to mimic the sport as much as possible.

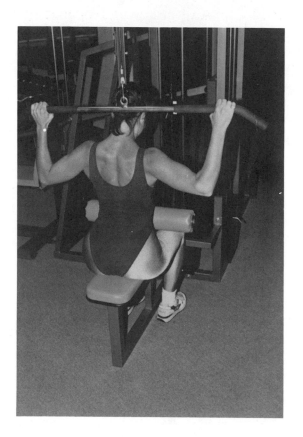

*Multi-station Gym*

## MULTI-STATION GYMS

Multi-station Gym machines can provide progressive resistance to almost any muscle group more safely than free weights. The training recommendations are basically the same. Again, if you are a beginner, start using a comfortable amount of resistance and gradually increase the weight.

For strength training with these machines, you can build up to six to eight repetitions comfortably. Then add resistance instead of adding to the number of repetitions. For endurance, use more repetitions at a lower weight. It's important to exercise your right and left muscle groups independently. If you always exercise both sides at the same time, the dominant group will end up doing more of the work, which will prevent the strengthening of the weaker side. Work quickly from one exercise to the next, to keep your pulse up. This will give some aerobic fitness while developing strength. And remember, always support your lower back.

## STRETCH CORDS

Elastic tubing or bands made of synthetic material or rubber are produced by different manufacturers to provide various forms of resistance training for both strength and endurance. Although the recommended programs and designs may differ between manufacturers, the principle of muscle work against resistance is the same.

**Pros:** These are some of the least expensive and most portable of all training devices. Their versatility allows for sport specific training for various sports. Some can also be used for flexibility training and low-impact aerobic workouts as well.

**Cons:** Sudden release due to breaking, slipping or releasing can cause injury. Remember, it's like a giant slingshot, and guess who's in the sling? If you have one end attached to the door and you're all stretched out, giving it your max at the other end, and someone opens the door...Bam! It's like the coyote in the Roadrunner cartoon, peeling himself off the wall.

**Helpful Hints:** So remember, get a good product that doesn't break or slip, and lock the door.
Some manufacturers offer a product with well-designed programs, even video tapes showing exactly how to use it safely and effectively, such as SPORT CORD[R] used by the U.S. Ski Team for training and rehabilitation.

The illustrations in this chapter are not meant to recommend specific brand names, but to give general guidelines for exercise equipment.

As mentioned earlier in this chapter, one of the most popular workout machines used by today's Indoor Athlete is the Stair-climbing machine. Besides providing an excellent workout, the Stair-climbing machine also provides insight into your entire fitness program. Just like on the Stair-climbing machine, the higher you climb in your day-to-day training, the closer you are going to get to your top level of fitness. And as we all know, **life sure is fun at the top!**

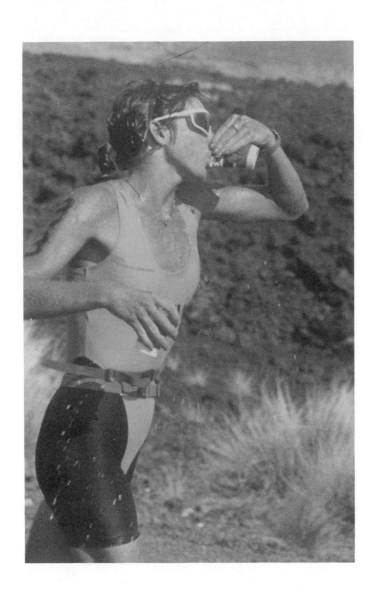

**Chapter Sixteen**
# Nutrition—Food, Fuel and Fluids

# Nutrition–Food, Fuel and Fluids

"Hey coach, where can I get some good New Trishian? I hear it's the secret to playing with less fatigue and lasting longer."

"No, listen, it's called good nutrition and it's not a secret. But if you don't know about it you better learn if you want to be there at the end of the game. Bad nutrition can cost you. It can cost you a first string position in the game of life."

> **nu-tri-tion** (*noo-trish'en*) **n. 1.** To eat correctly, to balance your meals, to provide the proper fuel for performance. **2.** To eliminate things like donuts, pizza, ice cream, french fries, etcetera.*
>
> **\* Etcetera:** includes anything and everything in the world that you ever enjoyed eating.

Now, now, things aren't quite *that* bad. There are still plenty of nutritious, good-tasting foods that you can eat on a daily basis. As you train, though, you have to start looking at your body as you would your car. If you fill it with lousy fuel... you'll get lousy performance.

## NUTRITION

Nutrition plays a vital role in the athlete's overall fitness and performance. The building materials that make up the individual cells in the tissues and the blood are literally constructed from the nutrients we absorb from our blood. In truth, **we are what we eat.**

Nutrition is also important to our mental as well as our physical well-being. If the food is of poor quality, the body won't have the materials it needs to build good, healthy cells, tissue and blood. It won't be able to function in a healthy manner, let alone perform well athletically. The body is constantly burning calories and breaking down tissue. In order to maintain the kind of burning and breaking down essential to fitness, the body requires a steady input of nutrients that will provide constant repair, growth and energy flow.

As soon as the body has a deficiency of the nutrients required to maintain the process of repair, growth, energy and performance will decline. Individual muscles and organs will begin to weaken and break down and illness may occur. Usually the earliest sign of breakdown is overall fatigue which happens more often than it should.

Nutritional deficiency can, at the very least, cause a drop in athletic performance and, at the worst, can lead to many illnesses. It is important not only to know what nutrients to ingest, but how much and when.

The days when athletes did well by just training hard are long gone. In order to stay competitive, today's athletes need to address their eating habits, sleeping patterns, emotional health, mental strength and much more. To effectively compete athletically, it is important that the body be carefully supplied with the appropriate amounts of essential nutrients at the proper time for peak performance. To do this requires awareness of what amounts, in what form, and at what time nutrients should be consumed. It is just as important to understand the digestive process as it is to understand what foods to eat. **You can eat the right foods but at the wrong time or in the wrong amounts and still not be practicing good nutrition.** The body won't get the fuel it needs and the results will be evident.

## DIGESTION

*Digestion* is the process by which we break down and absorb the nutrients we ingest. To improve the digestion process consider:

**1. Food quality—what you eat.** Try to use the best quality foods you can. Organic produce may be a little more expensive, but you'll save if you buy it in bulk. Organic foods are grown with no added chemicals—pesticides or additives. People who are concerned with food quality can no longer be called "health food fanatics." Nowadays, it is **wise** to know just **what** it is that you are putting into your body.

**2. Food quantity—how much you eat.** Overeating is one of the biggest causes of poor absorption from digestion and poor health. If the digestive system is overloaded, food will not be absorbed efficiently. This means you'll have less energy and exercise will feel "heavier" and more sluggish. Food is absorbed, but instead of being used for energy, much of it is stored as fat.

**3. Food frequency—how often we eat.** When we use food is just as basic to good digestion as which foods we use and how much we eat at a meal. The digestive cycle takes a certain amount of time. During the first three hours of the digestive cycle, 60-70% of the body's available energy is being used for digestion. If this part of the cycle is disturbed, there will be a higher energy output for the digestive process and yet a very low energy return because the digestion will be incomplete. Large meals should be four to five hours apart to allow completion of the digestion cycle. Healthy small snacks in between can sometimes be helpful without disturbing the cycles.

**4. Exercise after a meal.** Engaging in regular exercise greatly improves the digestion. Moderate activity after a meal, such as a gentle walk, also aids in digestion. But strenuous exercise–walking too briskly, running or swimming–during the first three hours can interfere with the digestive process.

When we do heavy exercise, more than 70-80% of our blood supply goes to working muscles, to deliver the enormous quantities of oxygen required. The first stage of digestion also requires a very large percentage of blood to be in and around the intestinal organs. **The body can't do both at the same time,** so the food won't digest well and the muscles won't derive much benefit from the training session. Fatigue will set in sooner and recovery will be delayed. If food must be taken just after or during heavy exercise, fruit usually works best. Fruit digests more quickly than other foods, with less energy cost, and provides quick energy for working muscles.

**5. Inactivity just after a meal.** Sitting for a long time, just after a meal, does not lead to overall good health. Lying down just after a meal is not a good idea and should be avoided. More food is converted to fat instead of being used for energy. Going to bed and going to sleep just after a meal is worse.

During sleep, your body shuts down in order to rest and recuperate. We can't sleep deeply and digest a meal at the same time. **Avoid eating just before bedtime.** Give your stomach two to three hours after dinner to complete the first critical cycle of digestion before retiring. The digestive system will absorb more nutrients from the meal, you'll get rest from your sleep and you'll have more energy the next day during exercise. Eating just before bedtime causes weight gain in most people, since more of the nutrients are converted to fat.

**6. Emotional calm.** Stress is not the situation in life that puts pressure on us. *Stress* is our inability to respond well to changing situations. There is definitely a correlation between stress and good digestion. Stress can be responsible for poor digestion, and we all know that excessive stress can cause ulcers and intestinal problems. That easy stroll after a meal is a good way to relax, slow down and aid digestion.

**7. Hot temperatures.** A hot bath, jacuzzi or sauna or resting in the hot sun after eating a substantial meal can lead to indigestion for some people. Your body can't maintain the first part of the digestive cycle and insulate you from hot temperatures at the same time.

**8. Fiber.** One way to markedly improve the digestive process is to ingest adequate amounts of fiber in the food. It has been shown repeatedly that people with a high-fiber diet have fewer intestinal problems and even less intestinal cancer than those who have low-fiber diets. The American Cancer Society recommends a high-fiber diet.

What is fiber? *Dietary fiber,* also known as roughage, is a carbohydrate found in whole grains, vegetables and fruit. Since it's not digestible, it is not broken down by the body's chemicals as it passes through the small intestine, and it stimulates the digestive tract. It retains water and adds bulk to the bowel movement. Studies have shown that fiber decreases blood cholesterol and fat. High-fiber diets have been shown to significantly decrease the incidence of colon disorders, including cancer.

**9. Chewing.** What do you associate with the word *chew*? Chewing gum, chewed out, chewed up, chewing the fat, chew-chew train? Or how about starting the digestive process off right by chewing your food?

Digestively speaking, there are two main purposes of chewing. One is to produce *saliva*. The action of saliva on the foods produces the first of several chemical processes in the digestive process. If the food is not chewed well and is too bland, an insufficient amount of saliva is produced and its chemical action on the food is incomplete. The other gastric fluids produced by other organs won't be able to do their work as well and digestion will be impaired.

One way to increase saliva is to make sure your foods are flavorful—but be careful not to use a lot of spices to accomplish that. Herbs are helpful and can make many otherwise bland dishes not only more attractive but flavorful and more fun to eat.

The other purpose of chewing is to grind the food into small particles so that the saliva and other gastric juices can thoroughly dissolve them. Even if healthier foods are used and properly combined and cooked, digestion may be impaired without proper chewing.

I remember when I was just starting high school, one of my good friends was a descendent of a great Comanche chief. At the time, he was a lot smaller than the rest of us and his father told him that if he chewed his food well, he would grow. Well, when Mom and Dad say, "Chew your food," most of us don't listen. But when the Chief said it, his son listened. He did just as his father told him. He grew, all right, tall but not fat. Now, I know that chewing can't make someone who is genetically small, large. But by paying attention to age-old eating habits, we can absorb more nutrients and have the best environment for the body to achieve its full potential. Our ancestors knew they must chew their food well in order to get the most out of it, and we know it today.

## THE FOOD THAT WE EAT

Now, what are the elements that make up the fuel we ingest? They can be broken into categories consisting of fats, carbohydrates, proteins, vitamins, minerals and water. These are the basic components of food. One way to balance your diet is to consume 20-25% fats, 60-70% carbohydrates and the rest protein, decreasing salt consumption to about five grams per day. (These guidelines are recommended by the government and the AMA.)

However, I find these guidelines difficult to follow when recommending a balanced diet to patients. Another way to put this is to say that the essential elements for an adequate diet are:

1. Sufficient calories to maintain the activity.
2. An appropriate mix of carbohydrates, protein and fat.
3. Adequate intake of fluids—water intake.
4. An adequate intake of vitamins and minerals.

**Calories.** Counting calories has classically been the way to determine how much intake we should have. If you're eating the recommended foods and exercising properly, you should not have to calculate the calorie count. Low-calorie diets have classically been failures—and mainly for one reason. If there are not enough calories, muscle is broken down. You may lose weight, but what you're losing is muscle—and you need adequate muscle tissue to burn the fat. It's a Catch-22.

**Carbohydrates.** This group of compounds is the central pillar for an optimum diet for the athlete, regardless of whether one is a marathoner, football or basketball player, surfer, skateboarder, or skier. In order to be able to train effectively, at least 60% of one's dietary calories need to be from carbohydrate sources.

Carbohydrate is stored as fuel in the muscle and liver as *glycogen*. During prolonged physical activity, these glycogen stores are used (predominantly the muscle glycogen stores). Inadequate amounts of glycogen can lead to a decrease in performance, speed and endurance. The amount of carbohydrates used is directly related to our glycogen stores. On the whole, complex carbohydrates obtained from breads, grains and vegetables are preferable to simple sugars for glycogen storage.

**Proteins.** Proteins are made up of amino acids. Protein is used by the body for building muscle as well as enzymes, hormones and elements of the immune system. Proteins are even used with energy sources in endurance activities such as long-distance running.

If there is a shortage of other energy sources, protein can also provide energy by breakdown. When protein is used as fuel, however, it is at considerable expense to the body, breaking down muscle and other important proteins. This breakdown causes more water loss and thus a false sense of weight loss.

In endurance activities, such as long-distance running, proteins are used as an energy source and account for up to 15% of the energy requirements. There is no evidence, however, that even with intensive training, more than 10-20% of the diet should consist of protein. Most Americans consume two to three times the recommended daily allowance (19/K per day). Too much protein can be a problem because it is not stored the same way as carbohydrates. Instead, its excess is converted to fat.

**Fat.** Fat contains about nine calories per gram as compared to protein and carbohydrates, which each contain four calories per gram. The fats we eat are usually divided into *saturated fats*, derived from animal products, and *unsaturated fats* derived from plant sources. It is recommended that two thirds of our intake of fats come from the unsaturated variety. It takes about 20 to 30 minutes of athletic activity before fat can be mobilized to provide fuel, so a workout of 30 to 60 minutes is needed in order to have any impact on the fat stores. I find it difficult to eat while using a calculator and a food chart, but it is important to know the basics. I recommend a diet that meets these needs but doesn't require a mathematical genius to follow.

**Hydration.** The importance of taking in adequate amounts of fluid is often ignored. Most people recognize the danger of losing large amounts of fluid, but what is often misunderstood is that even slight or moderate dehydration can effect one's ability to regulate body temperature and even stored glycogen. Adequate amounts of fluid are also necessary to eliminate the waste products from exercise. With more severe dehydration, muscle endurance and power are effected and even the ability to think clearly can be effected. A good rule of thumb is that an active person should drink about eight glasses of water a day, and increase this amount if intensity of exercise increases or if the environment is hotter or more humid.

Another helpful rule of thumb when exercising for more than a half hour, is to take in half a glass of water for every 15 to 20 minutes of aerobic exercise or for every three miles. Fluid replacement solutions that contain mineral and carbohydrate complexes are valuable, as they not only replace water but provide an energy source and minerals as well. Those exercising intensely, such as football players in pre-season camp, need to be especially aware of replacing their electrolytes. Solutions such as these are frequently used.

**Minerals and Vitamins.** Although popular belief would say differently, there is no good, scientific evidence that vitamin intake in excess of the RDA has any beneficial effect on performance. The same seems to be true of minerals. Very rarely will an active individual in the United States have a severe deficiency of either vitamins or minerals. However, people who exercise vigorously on a daily basis may need additional supplement above what they receive in their regular diet. Although this has not been shown in studies, the concept of taking a multiple vitamin with minerals on a regular basis seems like a reasonable and safe practice.

It is <u>not</u> true, however, that taking large doses of either fat or water-soluble vitamins is safe. Large doses of vitamins A, E,D,K (fat-soluble) for example, can be very toxic, as they are stored in the body. Water soluble vitamins such as C, $B_6$, Niacin, Folic Acid and $B_{12}$ can have serious side effects if taken in large enough quantities.

Vitamins do play a vital role in maintaining a sound diet. For example, the B vitamins help the digestive system break down carbohydrates, fats and proteins. Vitamin C helps form tissue in ligaments and tendons and protects against infection.

**Vitamin C.** Vitamin C supplements have long been controversial, since Dr. Linus Pauling claimed that large doses of vitamin C would aid against the common cold. Actually, moderate vitamin C supplements may cause no harm, since the vitamin is always excreted in the urine of the exercising athlete. It is even possible that a 500- to 1000-milligram supplement of vitamin C may be beneficial. However, there is evidence that megadoses (more than four grams of vitamin C) can be associated with kidney stones.

**Electrolytes.** This includes sodium and potassium and should be replaced appropriately if strenuous, prolonged activity is undertaken. This **does not** include taking salt pills. Solutions such as Gatorade$^R$, Recharge$^R$, etc. provide replacement in appropriate quantities.

**Iron.** Probably the most important mineral that needs replacement. For many athletes, both men and women, some form of iron should be taken as a supplement. The selection of a multi-vitamin that contains iron could be beneficial. But it must also be remembered that large doses of iron can be toxic and even moderate doses of iron can cause constipation and stomach aches.

# NUTRITIONAL SUPPLEMENTS

It is difficult to know what foods to eat, how much one should eat and whether to use nutritional supplements. Many over-the-counter products are advertized as key ingredients for successful athletic performance. Most of these have not been proven effective other than by anecdotal reports by their users or by taking information from studies and extending their findings to different situations. Does this mean that these products don't work or are harmless? The answer in many cases is that we don't know, because the appropriate research has not been done. Caution should be exercised, as using large doses of so-called "harmless" substances can be dangerous.

**Amino Acids.** These supplements are the building blocks of protein and have been reported as being the next best things to anabolic steroids in terms of muscle-building potential. The situation with these supplements is the same as with protein—there is no clear evidence that the athlete needs large quantities of them or that large quantities will stimulate muscles to grow. Large quantities of *anything* can be dangerous.

## THREE PHASES OF NUTRITION

Those involved in competitive sports should think of nutrition in three phases: Pre-event nutrition, nutrition during the actual competition and post-event nutrition.

**Pre-event nutrition:** This phase includes carbohydrate loading and what, when and how much to eat just prior to the competition itself. Carbo-loading is exactly what it says, that is, adding greater amounts of carbohydrates to the diet to increase muscle glycogen stores which should allow the athlete greater work capacity. Carbo-loading is only used for those involved in endurance events that can last more than one hour. People involved in sports like sprinting should not do this, as one retains 2.7 grams of water for each gram of glycogen stored —hence extra weight for no benefit. In sprinting, because of the short burst of energy expended, glycogen is not used as an energy source.

To carbo-load effectively and safely, maintain the normal carbohydrate diet (which may be 60-70% carbohydrate). Starting about two weeks prior to the event, the athlete should exercise more intensely than normal for about a week. Four to five days prior to the competition reduce the intensity of the workouts, but increase the percentage of carbohydrates in the diet to 70%. This has been shown to be safe and effective in boosting muscle glycogen stores. <u>Do not try to starve yourself while training to deplete your glycogen stores as was once recommended</u>.

In general, one should adhere to the following guidelines for a pre-event meal:

1. Don't institute new dietary practices the day of competition.
2. Allow enough time to digest the meal—two to three hours.
3. High carbohydrate foods with low fat and low protein content should be eaten.
4. Do not eat foods with high salt content.
5. Foods that have higher fiber content should be avoided.
6. Adequate fluid should be taken—one to two 8-ounce glasses of water.

If the athlete cannot tolerate a solid meal, try a liquid meal. There are nutritious products on the market which may be helpful, as they provide the above requirements in liquid form.

**Nutritional support during competition:** For events of less than one hour, water is the only requirement—approximately four ounces every 15 minutes. If the event lasts longer, a diluted carbohydrate drink containing minerals and electrolytes is beneficial.

**Post-event nutrition:** If you are involved in strenuous or vigorous activity, replenishing the carbohydrates that were used is very important. This replenishment must take place within *two hours* of the competition for maximum benefit. Nutritional liquid replacements or natural fruit or juice may be beneficial immediately afterwards—followed by complex carbohydrates later. The principles outlined here, in post-event nutrition, apply to training situations as well.

## ANABOLIC STERIODS

**Anabolic steroids** are compounds that are very similar to a naturally occurring male hormone, *testosterone,* found circulating in large quantities in males and in smaller quantities in females. They were first discovered to have strength and size-enhancing abilities in the 1950's. Since then, many athletes have used them and found that they gained in size, strength and ability to recover from strenuous workouts. These compounds probably work by preventing the breakdown that accompanies very strenuous, intense physical activities. Studies that show if anabolic steroids are effective have indicated that they only work in those exercising very intensely and who have adequate caloric and protein diets.

Many different types of athletes have used steroids, including weight lifters, football players, track and field athletes, body builders and wrestlers. Unfortunately, these drugs carry **serious** side effects, many of which are not measurable until severe damage has been done. **Many of these side effects are irreversible.** These include acne, effects on the heart, changes in sleep patterns, deepening of the voice, balding, increased aggressiveness and premature closure of growth plates in the long bones of children. The side effects are most severe in women and adolescents. Yet, no testing for steriods usage is done in the high school or grade school athletic programs.

Although many people claim there is a safe dose, this has not proven to be the case. Many athletes who take steroids take very high doses, as well as many different steroids at the same time. **These drugs are illegal, unethical and dangerous and should be avoided.** Many athletic organizations, both professional and amateur, recognize the use of these drugs and their danger and are beginning to enforce strict testing for them. Hopefully we will soon be in a situation where the pressure to take these drugs is no longer present. **Be cautious.** This is YOUR body—the only one you're going to have. Be careful what you put into it—not only **what**, but **how much.**

## WEIGHT LOSS

The important thing about diet awareness today is that it points to the fact that to reach better nutrition as a society we must decrease our intake of fats. This will require a major change in lifestyle. Fortunately, most athletes tend to be highly motivated when they learn what is needed to achieve a healthier body. The wise person will choose a diet that is low in fat, high in fiber. Guidelines should be set in motion to fulfill a long-term commitment to better health and to avoid becoming overweight.

An athlete who is presently overweight can reduce intake of certain fattening foods and consume only enough food to maintain body needs which translate to energy. When you reduce caloric intake, you achieve weight loss unless there is some type of medical problem and such cases are rare.

When considering weight loss, actual weight loss must be differentiated from water loss. Short-term weight loss is primarily water loss. **It comes back quickly.** The most important thing to consider about a fat reduction program is that fat loss is proportional to the energy deficit. Most nutritionists propose a balanced diet that consists of smaller portions of food with less fats and sugar.

Fat serves a very important function in the body. It is essential in maintaining body temperature and also forms a protective layer against harm to the vital organs. Fat circulates in the blood and is a source of energy for muscular contractions. There is a host of vital chemicals in fat that supplies the body with necessary nutrition.

## WEIGHT LOSS IN EXERCISE

The reason diets don't work without exercise is that **diets break down muscle unless exercise is part of the program.** Therefore, if you go on a diet without exercise, you may be losing a number of pounds but you'll be losing muscle tissue as well. Then, after the diet is over, you'll start taking in more calories. You have less muscle to burn the calories and you will store more fat with fewer calories than before the diet. The result: A few months later you end up fatter than you were before, because you will have proportionately more fat and less muscle than you did before your diet. Then you start this vicious cycle all over again.

**With less muscle, you'll do less exercise, become more inactive, and gain more weight on fewer calories.**

With regular exercise along with a healthy eating program, fat is burned during exercise and even after the exercise is over. With the increased metabolic rate established during the exercise program, calories are burned at a higher rate. Another benefit of exercise is that, since exercise improves mood and gives more energy, a person who is trying to lose weight will burn more calories because he or she will be more active.

One of the most important things in a weight loss program is the intake of water. The breakdown products need to be washed out of the system and you need plenty of water to accomplish this. When you exercise, fat is burned and muscle is built. Since muscle is heavier than fat, weight loss will not be significant. That's the reason I recommend that when you go on a prescribed exercise and nutrition program, don't weigh yourself. **Don't watch your weight. Watch your inches.** Watch the way you look and feel. Listen to the people when they say, "Wow! You're really looking good!" or "Hey, you've taken off a few pounds!"

## AN ANCIENT ALTERNATIVE

The *food classification system* has been used in several societies since ancient times. It's a more practical approach than the Four Food Groups system, because it demonstrates which foods should be used as Primary foods, Secondary Foods and Occasional foods. Under this system nothing is forbidden, but some foods shouldn't be used as often as others.

*Primary Foods* are the staple foods that should be used on a daily basis. A variety of grains, vegetables and legumes, nuts and seeds have formed the nutritional basis for most societies for centuries. The natural chemical make-up of these foods is neutral—not too much alkaline or acid, not too much sodium or potassium, etc. The further we've gotten away from using these basic foods on a daily basis, the more out of balance our blood chemistry has become and the more our health has suffered.

*Secondary Foods* are those foods that are good for our health, but that shouldn't be used as often as daily, primary foods. Their chemical make-up is a little further to one extreme or the other and, if used too often, they can lead to blood chemistry imbalances.

Depending on the individual's condition, activity habits, and climate, fruits and meats should be used only a few or several times a week, but not necessarily every day and certainly not with every meal as was formerly believed. Fruits can be eaten frequently but should not be considered a primary food source. They do not necessarily have to be consumed every day —and certainly not the same fruit every day.

*Occasional Foods* are usually those that don't contribute much to our health. Their make-up is so far from a chemical balance line that they can cause serious health problems if used too often. Most "junk food" fits into this category, and should be avoided most of the time, although it's all right to use them sometimes just for fun! Too much sugar (refined sugars, not natural ones like honey) and salt fall into this category.

## SUMMARY

1. Pay attention not only to what you eat, but when you eat, how much you eat and the quality of the food you eat.

2. Try to increase the amount of fiber in your diet. If you do not get an adequate amount of fiber in your diet through vegetables, grains, nuts and seeds and/or general roughage, then take supplemental fiber (Metamucil[R] without sugar or pure psyllium seed powder in small amounts). These help build the bulk of your stools and improve the digestive process. One of the most important sources of fiber is oat bran, since it has been shown to decrease the blood cholesterol. As you increase the fiber in your diet, <u>do so gradually</u>. If you're not used to much fiber, you might experience constipation or diarrhea, cramping and gas. Take it slow and give your body a chance to get used to it.

3. Adequate hydration is very important. Eight 8-ounce glasses of water is recommended. The more pure the water, the better it is for your body.

4. Have a balanced diet—low in fat, high in carbohydrates. Get most of your meats from fish and poultry. You don't have to abstain from red meat, but eat it in moderation, maybe once or twice a week, and then eat lean, high-quality meat. It's better to eat meat that has been raised without chemicals (hormones and antibiotics).

5. Next, look at your diet this way: Consider that a balanced diet consists of *primary* foods. These are the staple foods and should be used on a daily basis: grains, vegetables, peas, beans, nuts, seeds. This includes whole grain breads. Meat should be consumed, but not on a daily basis. Try to avoid "junk food." Anything that is high in sugar should only be eaten occasionally. Try not to add salt to your foods. You get enough salt in most of the prepared or canned foods you eat.

6. Don't eat the same foods every day. Certain theories on allergy show that a low-grade food allergy can be caused by eating the same food every day for a number of years. In fact, a four-day rotational diet is a good way to go. For instance, try to vary the grains you eat. We eat so much wheat in the typical American diet that it's a good idea to vary the grains—include oats, oat bran, rye and brown and wild rices.

Your body is yours, to do with as you wish. You can choose from a variety of foods and substances and decide what your body will get. The key word here is "choice," and the choice is yours. Have care and respect for your body and let your choices reflect this. Fuel your body in such a way that it will grow healthy and strong and in return your body will serve you and perform to the best of its ability.

As you can see, Nutrition is nothing new, but until we had seen, medically, the ill effects of poor nutrition, we did not truly appreciate it. Now healthy eating practices are being renewed. Maybe we should call it "Renew Trishian."

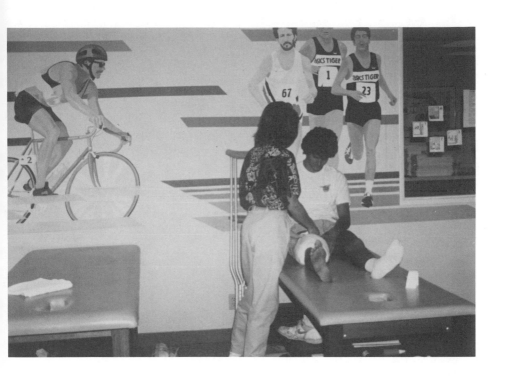

Chapter Seventeen
# Treatment

## Chapter Seventeen
# Treatment

Here it is sports fans. The Grand Finale. Everything you ever wanted to know about treatment of injuries in only a few short pages. Yes sir, from hang nails to headaches and more. My secret to the miracle cure for all sports injuries—simple straight talk—three magic words:

**Don't get hurt.**

But seriously, injuries do happen and they can be treated. So if you want to play sports and reap all of the rewards of being healthy and the excitement of participation and competition—Go for it.

Do what you can to avoid injury. And with the modern treatment available today, don't let the fear of injury keep you from participation and, whatever you do, don't let the fear of treatment keep you injured.

Injuries happen no matter what we are able to accomplish with education in the prevention of injuries. Fortunately, the range of treatments available today means that injuries can be less devastating than they have been in the past. Most injuries can be effectively treated either nonsurgically or surgically with the modern techniques available. The potential cause of future injuries can also be treated. When surgery is indicated, the technical advances that have been made in the field of orthopedic surgery allow most of the injured athletes of today to return to full-function in their sport. No longer is the active athlete satisfied when told to simply stop running because he or she experiences pain when doing so. Injured athletes often return to their sport physically stronger than they were prior to injury.

Getting to the source of the injury, the cause—and treating it with the same attention we have historically only given to the injury itself is the secret to decreasing future injuries and continuing participation. Frequently this is done through advanced techniques of physical medicine and rehabilitation, physical therapy and exercise therapy. For example, tendinitis is inflammation of the tendon. It is not enough to simply treat the tendinitis. We need to know what caused the tendon to become inflamed and treat that condition as well.

## THE SPORTS MEDICINE TEAM

Sports Medicine today is a team effort. Just as sports have evolved with specialized coaches, specialized training programs for special teams, etc., so has Sports Medicine evolved into a specialized team approach.

This team approach in dealing with sports-related problems has been effective and responsible for the great advances in Sports Medicine. Pooling the resources and talents of physicians of varied specialties (orthopedics, general medicine, physical medicine, etc.) with talented athletic trainers and physical therapists, exercise physiologists, podiatrists, psychologists, coaches, equipment managers etc., gives us the Sports Medicine team we need to insure healthy, active and more injury-free athletes.

The most important person—upon whom the entire team is centered—is the patient, the injured athlete. That person has the most difficult job of all—healing and making a comeback. Even while employing the best methods of treatment, without his or her active participation, the treatment program will most probably fail. It takes time, hard work, patience and confidence; confidence in the treatment plan, confidence in the Sports Medicine team and most importantly, confidence in oneself to overcome the injury.

### The Physician

After a four-year college course, four years of medical school and one year of internship, the general physician (M.D.) emerges, well educated in the latest knowledge and medical techniques. Afterwards, further study is possible if specialization is desired (as in orthopedic surgery, family practice, physical medicine, etc.) The orthopedic surgeon, for example, continues with four years of orthopedic residency. And this is often followed by further specialized training, i.e., Sports Medicine.

The orthopedic surgeon is trained to recognize and treat, both surgically and nonsurgically, problems and injuries to the musculoskeletal system. First, being a general physician, the orthopedic surgeon understands the body, overall, and its relationship with the musculoskeletal system. In this capacity, this specialist can work with the other members of the Sports Medicine team to serve the athlete to the best of his or her ability.

### The Team Physician

A team physician works directly with the athletic coach, the trainer, and the athlete to insure that the athletic program has the most up-to-date medical support available. Frequently, an orthopedic surgeon and a general medicine physician share the job of team physicians. The general physician attends to problems relating to general medicine. Together, they assess the medical needs of their team, while consulting specialists in various fields when a particular problem needs their expertise.

### The Athletic Trainer

Athletic trainers are educated to prevent athletic trauma and conditions which adversely effect the health of the athlete. They aid in management, such as first aid, evaluation of treatment, rehabilitation of athletic trauma and other problems that affect the athlete. The education and training required for athletic trainers is determined by state requirements and the requirements of their certifying organization (The National Athletic Trainers Association or the American Athletic Trainers Association).

The team trainer attends games and practices and often works as the equipment manager—fitting protective equipment and providing first-aid treatment. He or she identifies injuries and provides emergency care including cardiopulmonary resuscitation (CPR) and insures transportation procedures, until more definitive care can be administered. The team trainer is under the direction of the team physician and understands rehabilitation techniques and injury prevention.

And since the team physician cannot be present for all the athletic activities, the athletic trainer is indispensable. This is especially true since sixty-five percent of athletic injuries occur during practice. But unfortunately, less than ten percent of high school athletic programs have athletic trainers as part of their health care and athletic teams, leaving many young athletes without the expert care of this vital member of the team.

The athletic trainer also works directly with the coaches and the school program to recommend safe exercise programs designed for preventing and avoiding injury. The trainer is also a key link between the treating physician and the coach and between the athlete and the coach. The athletic trainer sets up conditioning programs for flexibility, strength and endurance which will help avoid injury. He or she will also advise the coaches regarding the safety of their playing facilities and their practice procedures.

More and more, athletic trainers are being utilized in capacities other than on the field. Today, athletic trainers are often utilized as assistants to physicians in Sports Medicine programs. In this role, they assist the physician and are able to provide an essential service to the patient by recommending training programs and conditioning programs that will help to improve the athlete's overall health. They are also used in rehabilitation in Sports Medicine clinics. In sports rehabilitation clinics, a team of athletic trainers, physical therapists, massage therapists and exercise physiologists pool their talents in order to achieve maximum results.

**The Physical Therapist**
Physical therapists are trained to relieve pain and expand movement. Training for the physical therapist includes four to six years of college, specializing in care and treatment, biological sciences, anatomy and movement.

One of the primary jobs of the physical therapist is to make sure that "the muscle gets the message." If the muscle is not receiving the proper impulses from the brain, then the affected area simply will not function properly. Proper movement cannot be restored and strength cannot be improved. Certain techniques are used to overcome this. Returning the function of the muscle is called *neuromuscular reeducation.*

Pain is the main reason why the muscle won't "get the message," since pain sensation will override the normal nerve impulse. This is called *reflex inhibition.* Therefore, one of the primary goals of the therapist is to decrease pain and therefore increase motion. This is accomplished through the use of various techniques and modalities employed by the therapist and the physical medicine specialist.

Certain physical therapy techniques have passed the test of time. The modalities of cold, heat and massage in treatment of injuries and pain have been used successfully as far back as the Greek civilizations. These are still being used today, only now we experience greater success due to improved, modern techniques. Modalities used to improve results include: cryotherapy (application of cold), ultrasound, and electrical stimulation.

**Cryotherapy**
Initially, ice minimizes swelling by causing a vascular constriction. There is less blood-flow to the injured area causing less swelling. This, in turn, slows the nerve conduction and decreases the pain in the area. By decreasing the blood-flow, the muscle spasms are decreased. This interrupts the pain cycle with the numbing effect of the ice on the nerves. Ice should be applied for about twenty minutes. Previously mentioned, R.I.C.E. means rest, ice, compression and elevation. The sooner the R.I.C.E. principle is applied to the acute injury, the sooner the swelling (edema) will decrease. The longer the swelling is allowed to occur, the more the body has to work to get rid of it.

## Ultrasound

Ultrasound is the application of high-frequency sound waves that cannot be heard by the human ear. These sound waves penetrate the tissue and may be reflected off the bone. This provides a deep heat treatment, removes pain and allows for faster healing. This can also help increase the motion of the joint by breaking up scar tissue and muscle spasms and decreasing inflammation of the area.

## Electrical Stimulation

Electrical stimulation is used in several ways. It can assist in decreasing pain and also in stimulating muscle contraction. A combination of electrical stimulation and ultrasound is proven to decrease pain and spasms, improving muscle function.

## Manual Techniques

Manual techniques used by therapists, trainers, and rehabilitation specialists, such as mobilization, massage and stretching, are helpful in returning function and reducing the muscle spasms. There are two basic types of stretching. One is the *passive stretch*. This is done by slowly putting a stretch on the muscle and holding it there for twenty to sixty seconds. This should not be severely painful but the muscle stretch can certainly be felt. The second type is a *hold/relax technique*. This method is based on the principal that after active muscle contraction the muscle relaxes and will be easier to stretch. This technique is best accomplished with a partner and is frequently used in therapy. It requires contracting the muscle against resistance.

## SHOULD AN INJURY OCCUR

Should an injury occur, then what? The injury is diagnosed and a course of treatment is prescribed. This may or may not include surgery. A rehabilitation program is designed for the specific injury and the patient begins the journey through the phases of healing and recovery until, once again, he or she is an active, healthy, injury-free athlete.

The goal of any treatment is to restore the body to full function as soon as possible by the most effective means. This requires cooperation between the Sports Medicine team and the athlete. Following any injury, there must be a span of time allowed for complete healing. It may mean dropping out of a game for ten minutes or as long as six months. All injuries require time to heal. They require the effort of the Sports Medicine team and the willingness of athletes themselves. Through modern techniques the team uses every means possible to facilitate the injured athlete's healing. And with the help of the athlete—healing takes place.

There are many ways that athletes can be active participants in the healing game. Given the right guidelines, the athletes should make their treatment process a positive experience. Not only is time involved in healing the injury, but the treatment program must be well planned.

No two injuries are exactly alike. Proper assessment of the problem and communication between the members of the Sports Medicine team is essential. Appropriate initial treatment may include casting, bracing or surgery, depending on the injury. Physical therapy is usually necessary for proper rehabilitation. Assessment and planning of treatment should also include psychological preparation for the patient. It is important in the healing process to consider the mind/body connection so that treatment can be a positive experience. After the treatment process the patient should be in better overall condition than prior to the injury, and thus able to help prevent injury in the future.

The first and primary goal of the rehabilitation program is to stop pain. This needs to happen in order for mobility, strength, flexibility, balance and coordination to be fully restored, thus helping to prevent further injuries. Pain is present with all injuries and an understanding of pain, and how it effects the body following an injury and during recovery, is helpful to the patient.

## FOLLOWING AN INJURY

Pain is one of the warning signs that usually sends people to a physician for treatment, but it is perceived differently by each individual. The pain can only be felt and described by the person experiencing it. And since it may be described in many different ways, it is the job of the Sports Medicine team to translate this description into a working diagnosis. It is important to consider the pain cycle and how it effects the individual and make one of the goals of rehabilitation to break this cycle.

The *vicious cycle* is associated with pain. It can best be described when the painful injury causes the muscles not to function properly. When this occurs, then there is less motion in the joint. The reduced joint motion causes the muscles to be used less, causing the muscles to get weaker. Any movement of the joint then causes more pain and thus more weakness. Add to this vicious cycle the psychological aspects of depression. The less movement and lack of improvement in function, the more depression, and the more the body chemistry is altered toward the negative side. While in the vicious cycle, recovery is difficult and doubtful. With proper treatment, however, this cycle can be interrupted. By breaking up the vicious cycle of pain and improving function, the patient can then move on to what I call the *vital cycle*.

In the vital cycle, there is a decrease in pain and an increase in movement resulting in an improved attitude with improved strength and, therefore, increased joint motion. Once the patient is involved in the vital cycle, recovery is almost certain.

The body's reaction to injury is pain and the body's response to pain is generally automatic. Its response may be to create a reflexive muscle spasm. This is the body's automatic way of protecting the injured area. This spasm prevents motion and further damage. With these protective spasms, the constant muscle contractions, or splinting, result in muscle fatigue. This decreases the blood supply to the muscle. The muscle will then adaptively shorten, restricting motion, causing another source of pain which occurs when movement is attempted. In this situation, muscles will become weak and other muscles will then substitute for the painful muscle, causing an adaptive type of motion. This motion is inefficient, and causes more injury to the effected area. Poor muscle coordination and lack of muscle strength can then cause further damage to the joint when the joint is moved in this weakened state. Utilizing modern medicine and the talented hands of the therapist, pain is decreased, the spasms quieted, and the joints are then moved, gradually increasing the range of motion to a safe level, not exceeding the body's normal range of motion.

## WHEN SURGERY IS NECESSARY

As a Sports Medicine orthopedic surgeon, I see many injured athletes. Most of these patients are able to be successfully treated and returned to their activities without surgery. Sometimes, however, injuries occur in which proper function of the injured area cannot be restored unless the involved tissues are surgically repaired or reconstructed. It is in these cases that surgery is recommended. Following surgery, it is essential that a well-planned program of physical therapy and rehabilitation be instituted as soon as healing will allow. This includes both physical therapy and a Home Exercise Program.

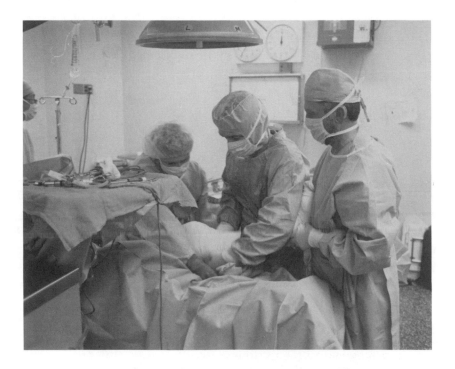

## REHABILITATION AND RECOVERY
## "WHAT TO EXPECT"

The goals of rehabilitation are:
1. To stop all pain
2. To regain mobility
3. To regain strength and flexibility
4. To restore balance and coordination
5. To prevent further injuries

When patients are injured, they should know what to expect during recovery. Recovery from injury frequently happens with a cycle of highs and lows. As patients are recovering, they will go through periods of time when they feel much better, and other times when they experience discomfort again. These highs and lows are not only acceptable, they are the natural pattern of healing and recovery. Although the rate of recovery is different from one individual to another, most everyone should expect the highs and lows that will occur along the way.

If you have a low back problem, for example, you shouldn't necessarily expect to feel less and less pain each day. If you do, that's great, but if you don't, don't become discouraged. Assuming you're receiving the appropriate treatment and therapy, you should begin to feel better after the first few days or weeks. Then, you could possibly have a sudden flare-up of pain. At this point, you may have a tendency to feel discouraged, as though you're back to "square one," when chances are you're actually progressing as you should.

One way of measuring recovery from an injury would be to look for these things as the weeks go by:
1. Pain episodes will be further and further apart
2. Pain episodes don't last as long
3. Pain episodes will not be as intense

If patients understand this natural pattern of recovery they can then avoid the common pitfall of feeling discouraged if periodic discomfort returns. Remember that the gradual reduction of pain will follow a pattern of "two or three steps forward and one step back." Continue with your therapy, your exercises, and a good attitude, and the goal of full recovery will be reached.

# THREE PHASES OF RECOVERY

In addition to the highs and lows that should be expected along the way, the recovery process has some distinct phases that will most likely be passed through.

*Phase One*—The Painful Phase
This is the period of acute or chronic pain. During this phase, the patient hurts almost all the time. There may be temporary relief from pain, but the pain always returns in full force. The goal here is to reduce pain and start to improve function. This can be achieved through appropriate treatment, sometimes including surgery. R.I.C.E., stretching, medication and ultrasound are some of the treatments utilized in this phase to reduce pain and initiate recovery.

*Phase Two*—The Pain-Free Phase
During this phase, treatment has reduced or eliminated the pain altogether. But full strength has not yet returned. This is the most dangerous phase of the process because "out of pain does not necessarily mean completely recovered."
During this phase, the injured area is protected with a brace, splint or cast. The tissues involved are not yet strong and stable, but since pain is decreased or gone altogether, there is a tendency to make two mistakes:

1. To give up the treatment that got the patient out of pain
2. To prematurely engage in activities that will worsen the condition (sports, lifting, too much work, etc.)

Either mistake will usually land the patient back in Phase One—The Painful Phase. Some people go back and forth between Phase One and Phase Two for several months or even years, when they could fully recover in just a few months if they only knew that, "Out of pain doesn't always mean all better." Be smart! Be a patient patient. Keep up the treatments and therapy and your Home Exercise Program that eliminated your pain and avoid questionable activities until you complete Phase Three.

*Phase Three*—Full Recovery

This is the phase in which the once-injured area is pain-free and the tissues involved are once again strong and stable. This means that the healing phase is complete. This is the re-entry phase. At this point training can be re-instituted, but with professional guidance. Depending on the extent of the injury and the time involved in getting to Phase Three, the patient will require training and conditioning prior to his or her entry into a sport, along with a Home Exercise Program including sport-specific exercises. Re-entry time can vary from several days to several weeks.

Also, by this time the patient should have a full understanding of why the injury happened in the first place. Perhaps it was a result of weakened postural muscles, coordination failure, or doing too much too soon. Learn from the injury and hopefully the Home Exercise Program will lead to a lifetime program of being fit, staying in condition, and avoiding injury in the future.

## HOME EXERCISE PROGRAM

This is the exercise program designed by the Sports Medicine team for the patient to do at home. This is a very important part of the treatment program. Here the patient has the opportunity and the reasponsibility to take a physically active role in treatment and healing. Through commitment on the part of the patient, the Home Exercise Program can extend well past the recovery phases and develop into an active life-long program to help insure a fit, conditioned and more injury-free body.

## THE ATHLETE'S RESPONSIBILITY

Ultimately, the recovery is the responsibility of the involved athlete. The athlete must be responsible for his or her own well-being and healing. It is important to follow the direction and instruction of the Sports Medicine team and comply with the Home Exercise Program. The majority of the strengthening and flexibility gains will be made through this program, which is entirely the responsibility of the patient.

## GUIDELINES FOR IMPROVING THE RESULTS OF TREATMENT AND REHABILITATION

1. Accept the injury.
2. Seek professional help immediately.
3. Educate yourself about the injury and treatment.
4. Be in good physical and mental shape prior to the injury.
5. Continue some form of exercise during the treatment—Be loyal to the Home Exercise Program designed for you by your Sports Medicine team.
6. Make it your goal that when treatment is completed, you will be stronger than before your injury and/or surgery.

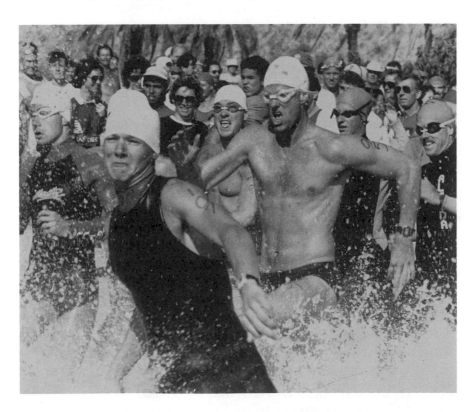

*When you're ready, "Go for it!"*

# Conclusion

This book is meant to be a guide that will affect the reader in a positive way. But certainly this book cannot take the place of a good physical examination by your health professional. If you have had previous injury, or you develop pain during exercise, seek medical attention early. Use the book to help you identify and understand your injury, but don't become your own physician. Let the professionals take care of you. There is an old saying among physicians..."A doctor who treats himself has a fool for a patient and a fool for a doctor." Anyone with medical problems should get a checkup before beginning an exercise program. After clearance from your physician, make his life easier by making fitness a part of yours and join the ranks of the Everyday Athlete.

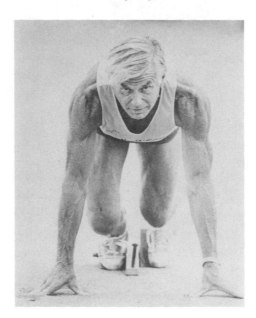

Remember, one of the hardest things to do after an injury, or after years of non-activity, is to **start**. So get into the starting blocks and get set to go for the best years of your life with fitness and exercise.

# Index